Understanding Dementia

Understanding Dementia

The Man with the Worried Eyes

Richard Cheston and Michael Bender

Jessica Kingsley Publishers
London and New York

First published in the United Kingdom in 2003
by Jessica Kingsley Publishers Ltd
116 Pentonville Road
London N1 9JB, England
and
29 West 35th Street, 10th fl.
New York, NY 10001-2299, USA

www.jkp.com

Second impression 2000
Third impression 2003
Fourth impression 2004

Library of Congress Cataloging in Publication Data
A CIP catalog record for this book is available from the Library of Congress

British Library Cataloguing in Publication Data
Cheston, Richard
Understanding dementia : the man with the worried eyes 1. Dementia 2. Dementia – Patients
– Psychology 3. Dementia – Patients – Care
I. Title II. Bender, Michael, 1943
362'1'9683

ISBN 1 85302 479 1 pb

Printed and Bound in Great Britain by
Athenaeum Press, Gateshead, Tyne and Wear

For Leslie and Molly Cheston
To Alison and to Gill

Contents

Part Three: Applying the Person-focused Approach to Psychological Interventions and Services for People who have Dementia

Part Four: Looking to our Future

List of Tables

List of Boxes

List of Figures

Acknowledgements

We should like to express our gratitude to Kay Harding for all her backbreaking preparation of the many drafts; to Alison Bender for her editing; to Andrew Norris and his family for allowing us to meet at their house; and to Ron Burns for his support and encouragement. We are very grateful to Dr Graham Stokes for permitting us to quote extensively from his article 'Reacting to a real threat' (1997). Whilst we were writing the final draft of this book, we heard the sad news of Professor Tom Kitwood's untimely death. This book could not have been conceived of or written without his pioneering work. We draw on: Bender, M.P. and Cheston, R. (1997) 'Inhabitants of a lost kingdom: A model of the subjective experiences of dementia.' *Ageing and Society 17*, 513–532; Cheston, R. (1998) 'Psychotherapeutic work with people with dementia: A review of the literature.' *British Journal of Medical Psychology 71*, 211–231; in particular, Bender, M.P. and Wainwright, A. (1998) 'A model of the mind in dementia.' Paper presented at the annual PSIGE conference, Napier University, Edinburgh, 2 July, and summarised in the *PSIGE Newsletter*, October 1998, No. 66, pp.22–24 as 'Dementia reversing out of the dead end'; and Keady J. and Bender, M.P. (1998) 'Changing faces: the purpose and practice of assessing older adults with cognitive impairment.' *Health Care in Later Life 3*, 2, 129–144.

For permission to reprint copyright material the authors gratefully acknowledge:

Extract from *Scar Tissue* by Michael Ignatieff, reprinted with the kind permission of Michael Ignatieff and Vintage Books, London.

PART ONE

Contemporary Attitudes

The man had been referred by a physician for assessment as to whether he suffered from a dementia. His wife did all the talking, but as she talked he smiled and nodded appropriately. There was no evidence of disorientation in his short replies, but it was his worried eyes that the psychologist noticed most: they were fixed on the interaction between himself and the man's wife, desperately trying to follow it.

Two weeks later, after the psychologist had undertaken some diagnostic tests, it was quite clear what the diagnosis was. At the meeting with the patient and his wife he did not wish to give feedback, feeling that this was the referring doctor's responsibility. The man's wife would not accept this and behind her glasses, her eyes flashed their annoyance as she recalled the tortuous path from GP to medical consultant to psychologist.

Under this pressure, the psychologist framed the sentence 'It looks as if your husband might have Alzheimer's disease,' but as he started speaking, his voice tailed off and stopped at the word 'Alzheimer's'. She thanked him and looked very relieved, as if now at last she knew what it was that she was dealing with. As the psychologist left the outpatient clinic he could hear her informing her daughter of the diagnosis quite calmly on the telephone.

By her side, the man stood quietly.

Introduction

A time of change

Dementia is an awful illness. As clinical psychologists we work with people who have dementia and with their families on a daily basis, and can see from them how terrible this illness is. Our knowledge of this awful illness is also a personal one. The grandfather of one of us had dementia. His name was Leslie Cheston and he served in the ranks of the Gloucester regiment throughout the First World War, both on the western front and in the Balkans. As a sergeant he had rescued one of his officers under heavy fire, an action for which he was awarded the Military Medal.

In the late 1960s, Leslie's wife died of cancer. He was prescribed barbiturates to help him to sleep and cope with his grief, but in those days many doctors did not appreciate the addictive effects of these drugs. Slowly Leslie's health deteriorated and he became increasingly confused, at times being unable to tell the difference between what he had dreamt while heavily sedated and what had really happened to him. The doctors told his family that he suffered from a 'hardening of the arteries' which reduced the blood supply to his brain. Today he would almost certainly be diagnosed as having dementia of the Alzheimer's type. The focus of this book is that we cannot understand dementia simply in terms of the medical model, as the effects of damage within the brain. We also need to understand the other things that are happening in a person's life. For Leslie, the experience of dementia was also a product of the bereavement that he had suffered and of his use of tranquillisers.

After some time living with his son, daughter-in-law and their young family in Norfolk, Leslie moved back to a hospital near Bristol, where he died a few years later. He was a brave and dignified man who was beaten down by the illness and by the inability of the services then available to him to understand his pain and grief.

This is a book about people who have dementia. Our aim is to help the reader understand:

- how the popular and medical concepts of dementia have developed
- the model that currently dominates research and practice
- what the weaknesses of this model are, and in particular how it encourages the subjective experiences of the person with dementia to be viewed as almost irrelevant
- another way of thinking about dementia, which takes as its starting point the subjective experiences of sufferers
- our own ideas of how we can best help people with dementia to cope.

This book has been written for people who want to understand dementia. It is most likely that they work in settings where they come across people so diagnosed or that they intend to work in such settings. Although we wished to write a book that was understandable and readable, we have used quite a number of academic references to support our arguments. We hope these will not put off the reader who only wants to use the ideas.

We hope that by the end of this book we have persuaded you to agree with two central ideas. First, we believe that to understand a person diagnosed as having dementia it is necessary to focus less on the diagnosis and more on seeing and understanding *the person*, their life and their experiences. Second, we hope to show that while we do not know whether dementia is untreatable, we know that, to date, it has been untreated. This is not to say that dementia may be curable – we will leave such claims to medical and genetic researchers – but only that until the last ten years or so, very few ways of working with dementia sufferers had emerged. The last part of this book will examine some of the psychological techniques, social and individual, that might form the basis of such treatment.

We also hope that by the end of the book the reader will understand the forces – cultural, academic and economic – that have shaped thinking on and research into dementia, and that they will feel there are more fruitful approaches. From such approaches may come more useful ways of trying to communicate with and help people so diagnosed, so that even if, as seems likely, the condition or more accurately conditions remain incurable, they are not untreatable. We can limit the damage and allow people to enjoy their lives for longer; it is our hope that this book will help the reader, wherever they work, to feel more able to achieve this.

For the worker in the field of dementia, these are interesting times. After the near-complete lack of interest of the 1970s, the end of the 1980s and particularly more recently have seen an explosion in the number of books and papers on research and practice in the subject. This work has progressed in a number of directions. Much has been concerned with the continuing search for an organic basis for dementia and the related quest for suitable pharmaceutical interventions, but we have also seen the introduction of social psychology and psychotherapeutic ideas into the field. These ideas have physical and human expression in the setting up of units such as the Dementia Services Research Unit at Stirling University and the Bradford Dementia Research Group.

Obviously, we consider that some of the developing ideas have more promise than others. In the second half of the book, we look at an approach which focuses on the perceptions and feelings of the person with dementia. Having elaborated on such a model, we discuss its implications for service delivery.

This book has a simple structure. Part One describes the existing framework – the standard paradigm of dementia; Part Two describes psychological ideas relevant to understanding the identity and position of a person with dementia in our society; Part Three applies the theoretical ideas outlined in Part Two to clinical work and describes therapeutic and service-delivery approaches that we believe are beneficial for people with dementia; and in Part Four, we look at what the future may hold.

This book will hopefully provide you with the tools to be independently critical of what you are told about dementia. In order to reach this point, you need to know what the orthodoxy is and what its limitations are. This is the purpose of Part One.

We start with a historical account of the 'discovery' of dementia. Part of the power of the present model is that it relies on an attractive myth: the narrative of the great scientist Alois Alzheimer making an important discovery, and then of medicine advancing by accepting this momentous discovery and steadily building on it. The reality – as detailed in Chapter 1 – is quite different. For this reason, we start by returning to the beginning of the century and Dr Alois Alzheimer's original work; we then describe how dementia went underground for some sixty years before being triumphantly 'rediscovered'.

The current orthodoxy builds on this myth. The organic explanation of dementia is essentially one in which parts of the brain are thought either to be dead or to have malfunctioned, directly causing the person's difficulties. So Chapter 2 offers a pretty straightforward and, we feel, balanced account of this model, and introduces the major subtypes of dementia – Alzheimer's, multi-infarct, Lewy-body and so on. The reader may prefer to start with this chapter and then go back to the historical perspective.

The organic model of dementia is dominant to an amazing extent. When we say 'amazing', this is because for any other type of mental illness there are numerous explanations, co-existing to a greater or lesser degree cheek by jowl. With 'schizophrenia', you can choose between genetics, experience in infancy, family dynamics, social conditions, brain pathology etc. Not so with the concept of dementia – the agreement between workers in various disciplines as to the validity of the organic model has until recently seemed to be nearly complete, and certainly was up to the end of the 1980s.

It might seem that the weaknesses of the organic model of dementia are of academic concern only, with precious little relevance to the day-to-day problems of people caring for and working with dementia sufferers. After all, at the point of writing, many great promises of rapid advances are being made, with the hope of a cure for dementia being held out by both genetic researchers and biochemists. During the lifetime of this book, a pill may come onto the market that slows down the progress of dementia. However, far from undermining the usefulness of the ideas that we are putting forward here, we feel that such a development would actually serve to increase the importance of our position. Such a pill would be a practical advance but would tell us little about what is actually happening in the mind of a person with dementia. The slowing down of the process of dementia by enhancing the person's remaining cognitive capacity would make it more important for us to have a detailed understanding of what is happening for that person.

In Chapter 3 we show that the organic model of dementia has very direct implications for the way a person diagnosed as having dementia is treated; we then go on to examine the effect of the organic model on contemporary treatment and services, and begin to highlight the deficiencies of such services.

In Chapter 4 we go over the various problems with the organic model. Here we must acknowledge our great debt to the social psychologist, Tom Kitwood, who in a series of papers (collated in Kitwood 1997b) became one of the first British psychologists to examine the organic model closely and describe various rather serious faults. Since then quite a number of writers have made other criticisms. Even neuro-psychologists working within an organic framework such as Hart and Semple (1994) have pointed out problems with the model.

Our criticisms of the standard organic model should not be taken as suggesting that psychotherapists are keen to work with people with dementia but have been prevented. Sadly this has not been the case. In Chapter 5 we look at the general resistance among the various schools of psychotherapy to working with the less intelligent or less socially acceptable members of society, which of course includes older adults and most definitely includes older people diagnosed as having dementia.

By the 1970s, some new approaches aimed at helping people with dementia were being introduced. The most important of these were Reality Orientation and Reminiscence. In Chapters 6 and 7 we look at the philosophy behind these treatments.

The second part of this book takes a significantly different tone to the first. In the first section we describe the current, largely medical, view of dementia that has shaped the provision of services and put forward criticisms of this model. The second section, by contrast, is concerned with work which uses a different philosophy – that of the new culture of dementia care. In Part Two we try to develop an understanding of the person with dementia as an active and interactive being operating within a social context.

We start by introducing the need to focus on the feelings and beliefs of the person with dementia rather than the views of a relative or a professional. We propose an approach that is psychological rather than organic, and which looks at the experience of dementia as that of a troubled person rather than a diseased brain. Chapter 6 introduces this person-focused approach and describes how people with dementia struggle to maintain their identities and develop coping strategies that are formed from and by their diminished cognitive abilities.

We try to make sense of the person who has been diagnosed as having dementia. One way of doing this would be to go back to undergraduate psychology, where students are taught that behaviour is a response to what is going on in the environment. In general psychology this is taken for granted, but the organic model, by making a direct link between brain pathology and behaviour and lacking any concept of 'mind', has tended to minimise this. Once we see those with dementia as people and not as diseased brains then it makes sense to look at the pressures to which they are responding.

A person – whether they have dementia or not – does not exist in isolation but in a social context. Having dementia and being labelled by others as such has a great influence on that context. The person with dementia has to handle and live in that context. So in Chapter 7 we look at the social context of being a person who knows they have and is known by others to have dementia.

We live in a system of expanding circles. Domestic life takes place in small, often family, groups; we have friends and acquaintances that we meet and communicate with; and most adults go to work and so have positions that carry with them expectations and responsibilities. Throughout our lives we also interact with large, somewhat impersonal organisations such as schools, social security and hospitals.

The person with dementia is likely to be over 65 and therefore retired. The range of facilities and the organisations that older people have to cope with and make sense of is rather different from those that a younger adult in work comes into contact with. The range of organisations an ill person – especially an ill older person – comes into contact with is again rather different.

There are also social pressures and attitudes that we need to handle. In our society being gay, being black or being a single mother are not neutral roles. The people inside those roles have to face various strongly-held attitudes that are expressed directly in the media and indirectly through welfare benefits and legislation. In the same way, the old are subjected to much negative stereotyping as asexual, slow, frail, moralistic, out of touch and so on; and the person who has been diagnosed as having dementia is the subject of still more and still stronger negative beliefs. The impact of these negative stereotypes is compounded by the fact that they are internalised and accepted as correct by many old people.

Armed with ways of understanding the individual's perception and the individual in the social context, we can look at psychological variables and processes that may contribute to disorientation. We see the loss of major roles that happens in old age, especially to women, as a key variable.

In Chapter 8, having described processes that augment disorientation, we look at how the difficulties that arise in the way in which a person processes information is a central feature of dementia. In the second half of the chapter we look at two models of the high levels of anxiety and bizarre beliefs that centre around the need for security that can occur as the severity of the dementia increases. The first theory, using information-processing ideas, concerns the frequent arousal of the person's Safety System – a rapid-response system designed to ensure their safety; the second is attachment theory, which has, in recent years, been applied to the field of dementia by the Dutch psychogerontologist Bère Meisen.

In Chapter 9 we explore further the emotions likely to be experienced by a person as they become aware of and concerned about their difficulties. We start by considering the emotions of grief, depression, anxiety and terror, and then move on to look at the coping mechanisms used to retain some measure of identity.

In Chapter 10 we examine the concepts of identity and position. We look at ways of maintaining position, such as becoming the person others take us for, keeping up appearances, and creating and maintaining identity through storytelling. Moving towards Part Three, this chapter introduces clinical material to show that people with dementia can reconstruct and re-frame their changed lives to gain or regain control in positive ways. This is the process of identity management, through which those with dementia are able to hold on to a sense of themselves as continuing to be essentially the same people that they always were.

In Part Three, we hope to demonstrate the usefulness of the person-focused approach. We also discuss its implications for service delivery and the assessment and treatment of people diagnosed as having dementia. In Chapter 11 we outline some general principles that we think should inform all such work with people who have dementia.

The reader might – quite reasonably – think that the assessment of dementia is a neutral, benign affair, perhaps a cross between seeing your GP and going for an X-ray. We start Chapter 12 by looking at the mechanics of and interactions between contemporary assessment procedures. We show that they are both confusing and dehumanising, especially in that the main communication is usually between professional and relative, thus bypassing and marginalising the person who is actually being assessed. We therefore recommend a complete re-framing of assessment as the beginning of a longer-term co-operative venture between the mental health professional (and their colleagues) and the person who has or may have dementia. It is the person who has dementia who should be seen as the client of the health, social and voluntary organisations. It is only if the initial contact between the person who has dementia and these services is based upon co-operation and honesty, that we can set the scene for future beneficial therapeutic interventions.

The next two chapters look at offering therapy to people with dementia. The first major therapeutic task, discussed in Chapter 13, is that of helping the person achieve a degree of emotional security so that they no longer feel that their world is crashing down around them. We outline how this might be done at various levels of severity. The second major task is to help them maintain a concept of themself as a person of some worth and value – to maintain their identity. At the earlier stages of dementia, verbal psycho-therapy should be available; Chapter 14 outlines the various types of therapy that should be available before considering how we can help the person with dementia to maintain their identity as their ability to put their thoughts and feelings into words deteriorates.

In Chapter 15 we look at the implications of a psychological model for service delivery in the context of community care. This concerns the maintenance of people who want to continue living in their own homes, and also those in residential and nursing homes. How would a person-focused model of dementia affect the way such services are offered? How can we get the users involved? How should we evaluate and conduct research into such inputs?

In Part Four we return to the world of today – the world of money, politics and power. We describe the forces that are determining what is being offered to people living with dementia because these forces will, of course, determine what chance alternative approaches stand. Looming on the horizon is a strong push by the pharmaceutical companies to sell drugs that they claim slow down the dementing process. Whether these claims are true or false, what effect will the arrival of such drugs have on services for people suffering from dementia? Adding to this strict cash limits for Health and Social Services, what chances are there for different ways of looking at dementia and treating its sufferers?

We suggest that, sadly, the most realistic answer to these questions is that contemporary political and economic forces will ensure that psychological approaches to dementia remain peripheral and that people with dementia will continue to be under-stimulated, over-medicated, and served by overworked, poorly-paid and poorly-trained staff.

In the final chapter we look at ways in which you can further develop your ideas and practices for the psychosocial care of people with dementia. There has to be – we have to hold on to – an alternative vision of what might be and of what can be if we care about and value people enough, regardless of their degree of disability. Other groups of disabled people – such as people with physical disabilities, people with learning difficulties, and people who are HIV+ or have AIDS – have made significant advances in gaining good-quality services. So it can be done; an alliance of professional workers and the young-old population (those in their sixties and seventies) might well win more resources and better, properly monitored services for people with dementia, be they in the community or in institutional care.

We hope that, by the end of this book, you believe that there are viable and better ways of helping people with dementia and wish to implement them to the best of your ability where you work.

CHAPTER I

The Creation and Recreation of Alzheimer's Disease

Enter Frau Auguste D, enter Dr Alois Alzheimer

April 1906: On the Munich train drawing out of Frankfurt station is a man in the uniform of an employee of the Municipal Mental Asylum. He guards carefully a large container. We cannot see inside it, but he knows it protects a large jar, and in that jar, bathed in preserving fluid, is a brain, the brain of Frau Auguste D, who was admitted into the asylum on 25 November 1901. The admitting doctor who clerked her in was the senior physician, Dr Alois Alzheimer, who recorded her severely disturbed and disorientated behaviour.

Dr Alzheimer left Frankfurt in 1903 but, always interested in brain structures, had an agreement that when Frau Auguste D died her brain would be sent to him. By 1906 he was working in the Anatomical Laboratory of the Royal Psychiatric Clinic, Munich. That was to be the final resting place of Frau Auguste D's brain.

The findings of plaques and fibrules in the brain of Frau Auguste D were reported by Alzheimer at the meeting of the South West German Society of Alienists on 3 November 1906. Since Frau Auguste D is seen as the first written-up clinical case of dementia, we will start this book with a historical account of Alzheimer's life and work; we will then go on to look at whether there are any other explanations for the behaviours of Frau Auguste D. Staying with the chronological approach, we will then describe how dementia went underground for some sixty years before being triumphantly 'rediscovered'.

In this chapter we will therefore present an account of the way in which the disease category of Alzheimer's disease came into being. We hope to highlight that the way in which the concept of Alzheimer's disease was formulated has meant that certain aspects of the experiences of dementia sufferers have been emphasised whilst others have been ignored.

Such is the power of our need for explanations and wish for cures that we tend to see continuity in medical advance, interpreting medical history as an inevitable, incremental advance towards better methods of assessment and treatment. Once an advance has been made it will, it is thought, stay in the medical collective consciousness and be implicit in the understanding and technical expertise required for yet further advance. Yet there have been critics of this optimistic outlook, such as Goffman (1961; 1963), Foucault (1967) and Illich (1975), and although their arguments are well known within academic circles they have so far failed to have a substantial impact on the awareness of the wider public.

This chapter has three aims:

1. A key paper by Alzheimer examines the behaviour of a middle-aged, female patient, Auguste D, and explains her behaviour in terms of her brain pathology, revealed at post-mortem. We wish to consider whether there are alternative explanations.

2. To examine the process whereby, in the early 1900s, a disease or condition came to be named after Alois Alzheimer.

3. To examine the re-emergence and rise to prominence of Alzheimer's disease since the 1980s and the influences that led to this.

Table 1.1 Chronology for Alois Alzheimer's work			
Date	*Alois Alzheimer*	*Emil Kraepelin*	*Other people/events*
1855		Born	
1856			Sigmund Freud born
1857			Eugen Bleuler born
1860			Franz Nissl born
1864	Born 14 June		
1871			German Unification

Table 1.1 continued			
Date	*Alois Alzheimer*	*Emil Kraepelin*	*Other people/events*
1883	Finished school	*Compendium der Psychiatrie* published	
1884 – 1886	Studies medicine at Berlin, Wurzburg (with Kolliker, the histologist and one-time colleague of Kirchow) and Tubingen		
1888	Graduated Assistant Medical Officer, later Senior Medical Officer, Municipal Mental Asylum, Frankfurt-am-Main	Appointed Professor of Psychiatry, Baltic University of Dorpat	
1888	Graduates in medicine		
1889– 1905	Working with Nissl, who Kraepelin described as a 'brilliant technician'		
1890		Accepts professorship, Heidelberg	
1892			Senile plaques identified by Blocq and Marinesco in an elderly person with epilepsy
1894	Marries banker's widow, Cecilia Geisenheimer. They have a son and two daughters		
1895			Breuer and Freud's *Studies in Hysteria* published (usually taken as beginnings of psychoanalysis)
1898	Paper on senile dementia		Redlich describes miliary scelerosis in two cases of senile dementia
1900	Gives up hope of becoming superintendent and joins Kraepelin at Heidelberg		Freud's *Interpretation of Dreams* published
1901	Wife dies. Frau Auguste D admitted to Frankfurt Mental Asylum		
1903/ 1904	Becomes Kraepelin's co-worker at Munich. Lecturer at University	Accepts professorship at Munich	

Table 1.1 continued			
Date	*Alois Alzheimer*	*Emil Kraepelin*	*Other people/events*
1905			Einstein publishes *Theory of Relativity*
1906	Frau Auguste D dies on 6 April in Frankfurt Mental Asylum. On 3 November Alzheimer gives paper at meeting of South West German Society of Alienists about Auguste D		Fuller discovered 'Neurofibrillary bundles appeared in senile dementia.' Bleuler, in Zurich, starts applying Freud's ideas to schizophrenia
1907	Published paper of above – a novel combination of clinical and pathological factors		Fischer at German Psychiatric Clinic, Prague (Director: Pick) reports neuropathological findings in 12 of 16 cases of senile dementia and none in 45 cases of progressive paralysis
1908			Freud and Jung invited to Clark University
1909			Perusini reports on four cases of senile dementia
1910		Kraepelin reports on Alzheimer's disease in eighth edition of textbook *Psychiatrie* (2500 pages)	
1911	Long paper on Alzheimer's disease		Bleuler's *Dementia Praecox* or the *Group of Schizophrenias* published
1912	Appointed Professor and Director of the Psychiatric hospital, Breslau (accepts against Kraepelin's advice). Falls ill with tonsilitis on the train to Breslau		
1914			Start of First World War
1915	Dies of rheumatic endocarditis Dec 19, age 51		
1918			Nissl dies
1922		Dies	

Alois Alzheimer

Alois Alzheimer was born on 14 June 1864. He studied medicine between 1884 and 1888 at Wurzburg. His academic career spans the period from 1888, when he took up his first post as Assistant Medical Officer at the Municipal Mental Asylum, Frankfurt-am-Main, Germany, until his death in 1915 at the age of 51, when he was the Professor and Director of the Psychiatric Hospital, Breslau, then part of Germany (now Wroclaw, Poland). During this period Alzheimer published 19 papers not only on dementia but also on a variety of topics such as general paresis and epilepsy, and classification in psychiatry (Berrios and Freeman 1991, pp.123–124).

As a medical student at Wurzburg Alzheimer had studied under Kolliker, a prominent histologist (McMenemey 1970). Histology was at that time an emerging technique in which, through the use of histological stains, medical researchers were able to prepare slides of nervous and other tissue for later microscopic examination. This technique played a major role in allowing researchers to develop new understandings of the actions of diseases within the body. When Alzheimer moved to Frankfurt in 1889 he met Franz Nissl who, according to Kraepelin (1917), was a key figure in the study of brain tissue and with whom Alzheimer was to establish a mutually productive working relationship. Alzheimer's association with Nissl lasted for at least six years (McMenemey 1970). Together Nissl and Alzheimer developed and applied histological stains which illuminated the cellular pathology of the brain to an unprecedented degree (McHenry 1969; Beach 1987). Alzheimer thus had the stimulation of working with a pioneer in histology. He also had another advantage. He could indulge his interests because he had private means as a result of his marriage in 1894 to Cecilia Geisenheimer, a banker's widow (sadly, she died in 1901). This allowed Alzheimer to combine his histological studies with clinical work.

One of the most influential figures of the day was Ernst Kraepelin, who in 1888 had become Professor of Psychiatry at the small Baltic University of Dorpat, before moving on to professorships at Heidelberg (1890) and later Munich (1904). In 1895 Nissl joined Kraepelin at Heidelberg (Burns, Howard and Petit 1995, p.1). Eight years later, having given up hope of ever becoming the Medical Superintendent in Frankfurt-am-Main, Alzheimer followed Nissl to work with Kraepelin, briefly at Heidelberg and then at Munich. Alzheimer was not initially paid for his work, being able to afford this situation due to his private means. The incentive was that Kraepelin had created a new grade of 'scientific assistants' who, as researchers, were free to use the scientific facilities and equipment of the institute (Hoff 1991, p.49). This co-operation quickly led to academic success.

> Appreciating the significance of Alzheimer's ideas for his own understanding of scientific psychiatry, Kraepelin provided him with considerable extra space for his Anatomical Laboratory, situated on the hospital's third floor. Both the staff and technical equipment of this department were the reasons for its growing reputation as one of the leading research facilities for the histopathology of the central nervous system. Among other co-workers and pupils were G. Perusini, F. Bonfiglio and U. C. Cerletti (Italy), H.G. Creutzfeldt and A. Jakob (Germany) and F. Lotmar (Switzerland). (Hoff 1991, p.49)

The basic purpose of this laboratory was to provide the scientific understanding of organic changes in the brain needed to underpin a coherent system of psychiatric classification.

On 3 November 1906 Alzheimer presented a paper to the South-west German Association of Psychiatrists about a former patient of his at the Frankfurt Asylum. Frau Auguste D was 51 when she was admitted on 25 November 1901.

> She had a striking cluster of symptoms that included reduced comprehension and memory, as well as aphasia, disorientation, unpredictable behaviour, paranoia, auditory hallucinations and pronounced psychosocial impairment. (Maurer, Volk and Gerbaldo 1997, pp.1546–1547)

She never left the Asylum.

Frau Auguste D

In this section we want to look at Alzheimer's central hypothesis: that Frau Auguste D's disturbed and disorientated behaviours were caused by the plaques and fibrils he found in her brain.

We know a little about Frau Auguste D. Although Alzheimer's famous paper is less than three pages long in translation (Alzheimer 1907), the casefile has recently been found and its contents published (Maurer, Volk and Gerbaldo 1997). In addition, Frau Auguste D's brain was later subjected to a second biopsy and there is consequently a small amount of information about her in Perusini (1909). Let us consider what is and is not known about Frau Auguste D.

The absence of a biographical or social context

Alzheimer tells us nothing about Frau D's previous life. In neither the original paper nor the case notes is there any reference to the life history of Frau D. Her behaviours are all described in the here and now. There is no attempt to see any continuity between her present distressed state and her past, no developmental approach (Erikson 1985; Sugarman 1986). This way of presenting Frau D's behaviours contrasts not only with the contemporary writings of Freud in Vienna but with Bleuler's 1911 monograph on the behaviour of people that he described as suffering from dementia praecox (what we now call schizophrenia) (1950; First published 1911). The depiction of Frau D outside the context of a life story strengthens Alzheimer's explanation of her behaviour in terms of cellular changes occurring within her brain, as it is the only explanation available.

Alternative clinical explanations for Frau D's behaviour

Alzheimer begins his paper as follows:

A unique illness involving the cerebral cortex

A case report from the Mental Institution in Frankfurt ant Main

THE CLINICAL COURSE and pathology of this distinctive process separate it from the known neurological disorders.

The patient initially presented at fifty-one years of age with jealousy of her husband. Rapidly progressive memory loss soon followed. No longer finding her apartment suitable, she dragged her furniture back and forth and concealed it. She began to believe that others wanted to kill her, and she would scream out loud.

Following institutionalisation she appeared totally bewildered. She was disoriented as to time and place and occasionally stated that she did not understand events around her. She treated her physician as a guest, excused herself and said she was not finished with her work. Following this she would scream aloud that he was trying to stab her with a knife, or indignantly turn him away, fearing that he would violate her. She was intermittently delirious, dragged her bedding about, called for her husband and daughter, and appeared to be having auditory hallucinations. She would scream for hours in a monstrous voice.

She was unable to understand situations and would scream every time someone would attempt to examine her. Only after repeated attempts could an examination be performed. (Alzheimer 1977; First published 1907)

This picture is curious. Frau Auguste D seems to be repulsed by physical contact. We would certainly think that this is a woman in a psychotic state. Alzheimer apparently thought this case 'a peculiar form of senile psychosis' (Perusini 1911), but this woman was *not* senile – she died when she was 55. One might consider paranoia (the jealousy, the fear of attacks) or a psychosis induced by violent sexual assault ('she would scream aloud that he was trying to stab her with a knife'; 'She would scream every time someone would attempt to examine her'), possibly by her husband, by someone else, perhaps unknown to her husband, or by somebody her husband did not (wish to) believe capable of such behaviour. Interestingly, 80 years later Graham Stokes (1997) wrote up a remarkably similar case:

> Mrs O is a seventy-five year old woman suffering from a marked dementia of the Alzheimer type. Following the death of her husband several years earlier, she lived by herself until self-neglect and increasingly risky behaviour led to an admission into residential care. From the moment she entered the specialist dementia unit, she was a cause for concern. She was also a puzzle.
>
> In daily life around the home she rarely displayed awareness of her surroundings. She spent much of the day sitting contentedly, often smiling at passers by, nodding and occasionally gesturing with her hand. She would participate passively in activities, and conveyed an aura of kindliness. Yet, profoundly forgetful, grossly disoriented and lacking meaningful speech, she also had high dependency needs.
>
> Unfortunately, she reacted very badly to intimate care. At such times, she seemed transformed beyond recognition. Helping her out of bed, assisting her with dressing and washing were all met with unbridled ferocity. She was labelled unco-operative and violent, her behaviour dismissed as typical of advanced dementia.
>
> It was her toileting difficulty, however, that caused greatest concern. Despite being inappropriately labelled by many staff as incontinent, she retained bladder control. She was rarely found wet in her bed or chair. Instead she would be observed walking around soiled. Staff would find wet clothing hidden away, and on occasions she would smear her bedroom or toilet. Helping her in the toilet, checking to see if she was wet, and attempting to change her clothing caused Mrs O great distress.
>
> Her screams, abusive language and physical assaults on staff often degenerated into struggles. Two staff would invariably attempt to toilet

her. This made the situation 'manageable', but in no way reduced the trauma of the experience. Yet it was not her toileting difficulty that brought matters to a head. The catalyst for understanding was Mrs O's ulcerated legs.

Her leg ulcers had been a problem while she lived at home, and the district nurse regularly cleaned and dressed them. Mrs O appeared to have enjoyed these visits. Not only was there no record of distressed or unco-operative behaviour, but the notes documented how 'chatty' and 'jolly' she seemed. In the home, however, the senior care staff who now had responsibility for changing her dressings, were met with the same distress observed during toileting. (p.14)

In this case, an explanation was forthcoming:

While there was regular contact with Uncle H, Mrs O's elder brother, they rarely saw her younger siblings (two sisters and a brother). Whenever they did meet there was tension in the air.

Uncle H still figured in his sister's life. He often visited the home, and regularly shed tears. Staff would see him holding her hand, and would occasionally decipher the words 'I'm sorry, pet'. No other relatives visited.

One day I happened to visit the home at the same time as Uncle H. He had been particularly upset during his visit, and staff had comforted him in a side room. They asked whether I would speak to him, and our conversation uncovered the motivation for his sister's difficult behaviour.

I had expected to be counselling a man distressed by the sight of advancing dementia. But he started to rebuke himself for letting his sister down, not standing by her when the others turned against her. He had always known that what she said was true, for he had been there. For years Mrs O had been subject to sexual abuse at the hands of her father. Uncle H had known about it; so had his eldest brother (killed during the Second World War). Their mother was protective towards her daughter, yet also colluded with her husband's abusive behaviour. She ensured that the matter was never spoken about.

The younger siblings never knew, and they loved their father. So when Mrs O, consumed with guilt and self-disgust, confided in her sisters, she did not receive understanding and compassion. They accused her of being malicious, and eventually ostracized her.

Why Mrs O was abused and not her sisters warrants only speculation. Uncle H did say their mother once had a friendship with a man who lived in an adjacent street, and who appeared especially fond of Mrs O when she was a young child. Could this be the explanation? A love child who became a figure of torment, an unwelcome reminder of infidelity? (p.15)

Goldsmith (1996) describes another case where there were difficulties in taking a lady to the toilet: 'The staff found this a difficult and degrading exercise until we were informed that our resident had been raped as a young woman' (pp.129–130). Walker and Pinhey (1991) discuss other cases of this kind.

The symptomatic presentation of sexual abuse was not uncommon in this period of high-Victorian morality, unquestioned paternalistic authority and female subjugation. It was only a few years earlier, in 1895, that Josef Breuer and Sigmund Freud had published *Studies on Hysteria* (1955; First published 1895). Breuer was a friend of the physician Moriz Benedikt (Borch-Jacobsen 1996, p.67) and refers to his work in *Studies on Hysteria*: 'Benedikt says he cured an adolescent girl's hysterical symptoms by getting her to talk about having been raped at the age of seven' (Breuer and Freud 1955, p.210).

The main case presentation in *Studies on Hysteria*, the original statement of psychoanalytic thinking, is that of Fraulein Anna O, who was treated in Vienna but, coincidentally, came from Frankfurt (Borch-Jacobsen 1996, p.98). Here the clinical condition of hysteria is ascribed to sexual abuse, most often parental but also marital.

> It is surprising that the wedding night does not have pathogenic effects more frequently, since unfortunately what it involves is so often not an erotic seduction but a violation ... sexual traumas also occur in the later course of many marriages. The case histories from whose publication we have been obliged to refrain include a great many of them – perverse demands made by the husband, unnatural practices etc. (Breuer and Freud 1955 [first published 1895] p.246; see also Masson 1985)

In contrast, Alzheimer gives no credibility to Frau D's sexual concerns and fears. The case notes give no indication that he interviewed the husband (Maurer, Volk and Gerbaldo 1997). Of course, systemic ideas about family dynamics were many years in the future (for example, Handel 1968), and it is a measure of Freud's genius that he could, at least at first, contemplate the existence of parental sexual abuse. But with the benefit of hindsight we may say that Auguste D's behaviours were poorly investigated. For example, in the case notes, Alzheimer notes:

> When she was brought from the isolation room to the bed she became agitated, screamed, was non-co-operative; showed great fear and

repeated: *I will not be cut. I do not cut myself.* (Maurer, Volk and Gerbaldo 1997, p.1547; emphasis in the original)

If Frau D does not cut herself, then who did she believe was threatening to cut her? Had she had a painful episiotomy? Alzheimer continues describing her progress:

Her focal symptoms clearly waxed and waned; but they remained minimal during her illness. However her mental deterioration was progressive. (Alzheimer 1977, p.41; original 1907)

While Alzheimer gives no explanation as to why her focal neurological signs varied in this way, we should note that such variation accords better with a functional than with an organic explanation.

A further aspect deserves consideration. Given Frau D's history of five years in the asylum, what we now recognise as institutionalisation would undoubtedly have occurred (Barton 1959; Goffman 1961; Wing and Brown 1970). Moreover, if as was likely, Frau D was often placed in isolation, then she would have suffered from sensory deprivation and chronic under-stimulation. It is quite conceivable that over sufficient time both these conditions could have contributed to an irreversible decline in functional skills and the subsequent organic brain changes.

She died after four and a half years of illness. Prior to her death she had become completely apathetic, went to bed in her clothes, neglected her personal hygiene, and developed decubitus ulcers despite nursing care. (Alzheimer 1977, p.42, original 1907)

The end state description tells us little. On the surface she seems to have lost the will to live rather than her abilities, as Alzheimer does not say she was unable to dress or wash herself. Functionally, not dressing or washing, by decreasing her attractiveness, would decrease the chance of further assault. A lack of motivation to undertake these tasks rather than an absolute loss of the ability to do so is more indicative of depression than of dementia.

Using the rhetoric of scientific discovery

The standard account of Alzheimer's discovery is that he was a pioneer in discovering plaques and fibrils, and that these brain changes were the cause of Frau D's condition. Both are open to serious doubt. Certainly, his use of the Bielschowsky silver technique was a technical advance. With this technique, Alzheimer demonstrated the presence of abnormal fibrils and miliary foci or plaques – the two neurological changes that are now held to be almost synonymous with Alzheimer's disease. However, the existence of neurofibrils had been known about for some time, while plaques had been associated with dementia since the 1880s (Harding and Palfrey 1997). Relating plaques and fibrils to dementia in 1906, therefore, was not a scientific discovery or breakthrough.

Second, the most obvious change in Frau D's brain was *not* the plaques or neurofibrils; it was brain atrophy, and Alzheimer starts his description: 'The brain sections demonstrated generalised atrophic changes. The major cerebral vessels showed atherosclerotic changes' (Alzheimer 1977, p.42).

Atherosclerosis is a disease in which the inner layer of the arterial wall thickens. So, clearly, Frau Auguste D had two things wrong with her brain: atherosclerosis and the plaques etc. Alzheimer considered that it was the combination of atherosclerosis and the plaques that created the condition. It was only later that 'atherosclerosis was quietly dropped and became an exclusion criterion' (Berrios 1990, p.363).

Placing Frau D within a wider psychiatric framework

As we said earlier, Alzheimer thought this case 'a peculiar form of senile psychosis' (Perusini 1911). But Frau D was not senile – she died when she was 55. What Alzheimer was attempting to do was to argue that the behaviours associated with senility could occur at a younger age. For Alzheimer this was evidence in support of a continuity model of ageing.

> Alzheimer felt that he was describing a novel combination of clinical and pathological features, i.e., a form of dementia characterized by focal symptoms developing in a young patient with senile plaques and neurofibrillary tangles (although it is often forgotten that arteriosclerotic features were also present). (Burns *et al.* 1995, p.3)

While it is clearly impossible to do anything more than to speculate about the meaning and significance of Frau D's behaviour, it is important to emphasise that the evidence that Alzheimer used to deduce the organic explanation of Frau D's behaviours can be interpreted in a number of different ways. Aspects that need to be considered are:

- Alzheimer's autopsy showed both vascular and cellular changes. Accepting for the sake of argument the organic explanation of causality, it is unclear and unknowable how much or which of Frau D's behaviours relate to the arteriosclerosis and how much or which to the cellular changes.

- The apparent lack of agreement as to the major features of the post-mortem on the same brain as reported by two leading anatomists. Alzheimer reported two changes as affecting the brain of Frau Auguste D: arteriosclerosis and fibrilary plaques. However, later, in 1909, Perusini used Auguste D's brain again in an apparent attempt 'to accumulate evidence in favour of the new "disease"' (Berrios 1990, p.360). Like Alzheimer, Perusini was clearly an accomplished histologist. Yet Perusini's description differed in some respects from Alzheimer's report. For example, Perusini's post-mortem results made no reference to arteriosclerotic changes. Arteriosclerosis was dropped as a competing explanation for Frau D's behaviour and instead became an exclusion criterion. (Berrios 1990, pp.360–363)
- It is unclear *when* the reported brain changes took place. They could well have occurred *after* admission. In this case they would be causally unrelated to the behaviours that occurred before or at admission. Certainly, the sexual fears may well have been independent.
- The complete lack of information about Frau D's life.
- Alzheimer's lack of concern for the psychological meaning of her complaints.
- Insufficient information as to whether she was unwilling to carry out tasks (indicative of depression) or unable to (indicative of dementia).
- The effects of sensory deprivation and institutionalisation in depressing competence. (Barton 1959; Wing and Brown 1970)

The case of Auguste D has been held up as an elegant demonstration of the correctness of the organic explanation. In retrospect we can see that this is only true if the correctness of the organic explanation is assumed and used to frame the reading of the text.

Kraepelin's creation of 'Alzheimer's disease'

Alzheimer was not the only medical researcher to report behaviour such as that displayed by Frau Auguste D and ascribe it to neurological causes. Other researchers had described cases similar to Frau D: for example, Perusini reported four cases in 1909 (Burns *et al.* 1995, p.3) while Fisher described a longer series of 16 cases of senile dementia in 1907 (*see* Table 1.1). As Burns *et al.* (1995) wrote: 'We could just as easily be speaking about Perusini's, Bonfiglio's, Fuller's or Fischer's disease' (p.4). Berrios (1990) remarks:

Where was the novelty in Alzheimer's description? It is likely that all he meant to emphasize in his short report was the fact that a dementia of the senile type could also occur in a younger person. This is confirmed by what he said in the 1911 paper and by the commentaries of those who worked with him. For example, Perusini (1911) wrote that for Alzheimer 'these morbid forms do not represent anything but atypical forms of senile dementia'. (p.360)

The main reason why we now refer to Alzheimer's disease rather than to Perusini's, Bonfiglio's, Fuller's or Fischer's disease is because of Kraepelin's incorporation of the case that Alzheimer had described into his psychiatric textbook. In the eighth edition, published in 1910, he created a sub-type of 'senile dementia' called 'Alzheimer's disease', 'a particularly serious form of senile dementia' (Kraepelin 1910, quoted in Maurer, Volk and Gerbaldo 1997, p.147). Kraepelin thus interpreted Alzheimer's work on one atypical example as proof of a general disease process. Yet it does not seem likely that Alzheimer saw his case findings as being of great theoretical importance, as his paper is only three pages long and he did not write a longer paper elaborating on the case. Kraepelin, however, was less modest on behalf of his colleague and, indeed, there is some evidence that Alzheimer himself was both surprised and a little embarrassed by Kraepelin's attention (Burns *et al.* 1995).

In order to find out why Kraepelin championed Alzheimer's work, we need to understand that as the head of a large academic institution Kraepelin had to compete with other institutions for prestige and influence. At this time similar work was being carried out in Pick's laboratories at the University of Prague, most notably by Fischer, who undertook larger studies of patients and also used control groups. Other institutions were also working on the development of histological methods and the classification of illnesses. Many of the neurological conditions – such as Pick's disease (Pick 1906) and Creutzfeldt-Jakob's disease (Jakob 1921) – were first described around this time. Therefore, in claiming this 'new' disease for Alzheimer, Kraepelin was also claiming it for himself, for his institution, and perhaps most importantly of all, for his overall conception of mental illness, to which we now turn.

At the end of the nineteenth century, 'dementia' had a much wider and less focused meaning than it has today. It was used to refer to 'any state of psychological dilapidation associated with chronic brain disease' (Berrios and Freeman 1991, p.2). Part of the task that the academic psychiatry of that time had set itself was to break down this unwieldy conceptual lump into more exact terms, framing them within a scientific rhetoric so as to justify their use. Thus Kraepelin advocated close study of 'the course of the illness' in order to discover natural groupings (Boyle 1990, p.10). He hoped to put psychiatry and psychiatric classification onto a scientific footing by linking the clinical behaviours that characterised psychiatric illnesses to underlying brain pathologies. For instance, Kraepelin had earlier separated 'manic-depressive insanity' from 'dementia praecox' (a term which he borrowed from Morel (1852), who had coined the term 'démence precoce' to refer to a state of dementia during adolescence).

There was, at the time, very little evidence of such a correspondence between behaviour and brain pathology. The one much vaunted exception was General Paresis of the Insane, which had been shown to be related to the presence of syphilitic spirochetes. In order for Kraepelin to substantiate his claim that organic change within the brain was the prime cause of mental illness, at least four discursive practices were used. These can be summarised briefly as follows:

- First, as we have seen, the role of histological techniques was emphasised. However, whereas Alzheimer had described Frau Auguste D as an atypical example of premature senility, occurring as the result of two age-related changes arising within the brain of a woman in her mid-fifties, Alzheimer's disease, as described by Kraepelin, was a distinctive disease resulting from the action of a single process. Thus, despite Kraepelin's appeal to medical technology for evidence to support his conclusions, the disparate accounts of Perusini and Alzheimer show that this evidence also relied on subjective interpretation.

- Second, other similar cases needed to be located – a task that proved more difficult than one might imagine:

  ...the curious thing is that when Kraepelin baptized the disease (it is likely that he completed writing that section of the Handbook in 1909), only five cases had been reported. It is also of some interest to note that Perusini's (1909) first case (he reported four in 1909 paper) is in fact Alzheimer's first case in which some features have been changed (for example, the post-mortem results no longer showed arteriosclerotic changes!). Likewise, Perusini's fourth case (in the same paper) was Bonfiglio's (1908).

  It is an important question to ask why these cases needed to be re-reported. The answer is that probably there was great pressure in the laboratory to accumulate evidence in favour of the new 'disease'. (Berrios 1990, p.360)

- Third, Kraepelin argued that his findings were drawn from a study of 'the natural progression' of the illness. This concept of a 'natural progression' is a very odd one, since we cannot know what would happen if 'the illness' were treated by people holding different beliefs and using different methods – and the more damaged our systems, the more important the effect of the environment (Lawton 1980b). In short, the impact of the environment and the social system were almost completely ignored within this framework. As we have described above, Alzheimer was also working within this framework in positioning Frau D outside the context of either a personal history or the influence of social factors.

- The movement from the case of Frau D to Alzheimer's disease represents a transition from the personal and particular to the objective, general and high-status. This is a transition controlled by a man of high status and dependent upon the experiences of a woman of low status. Thus, in referring to this newly created disease as Alzheimer's disease, Kraepelin was able to distance himself from his creation, again lending weight to his analysis of organic psychiatry.

In conclusion, Kraepelin's representation of Alzheimer's discovery as a distinct subtype of senile dementia contrasts with Alzheimer's own account of his work, in which it is clear that he was describing a particular and unusual set of clinical behaviours and corresponding brain pathology, not a new brain disease. It seems clear that by depicting Alzheimer's account of Frau Auguste D in this fashion Kraepelin was seeking to lend weight to his own descriptive categories, and that it was Kraepelin, not Alzheimer, who created Alzheimer's disease.

The re-creation of Alzheimer's disease

Although Kraepelin had essentially created Alzheimer's disease through his incorporation of Alzheimer's study of Frau Auguste D into his textbook of 1910, it was not until roughly 70 years later that this disease concept began to attract the attention of psychiatrists, researchers and the general public to a significant extent.

It is important that the reader appreciates the discontinuity between the First World War and the 1970s. During this period there was almost no research into Alzheimer's disease whatsoever. Terry's 1963 paper using electron microscopy, in America, and the work of the Newcastle group (e.g. Roth, Tomlinson and Blessed 1967) can be used as end markers for some fifty years of silence and lack of interest. If we consider a well-regarded British psychiatric text of the 1960s and 1970s, Fish's *Outline of Psychiatry*, Second edition (1968), Alzheimer's disease is described as 'the commonest pre-senile dementia', and its description is confined to just one page (p.160). Similarly, if we look at an overview of dementia from that time, Miller's well-regarded *Abnormal Ageing: The Psychology of Senile and Pre-Senile Dementia* (1977), a book of 144 pages of text, Alzheimer's papers are not referenced and Alzheimer's disease is mentioned only five times. There is no detailed description of the disease, although there is a discussion of its differential diagnosis, which consists of two paragraphs. Maher, in his text *Principles of Psychopathology* (1970) summarised the current opinion: 'Alzheimer's disease is statistically infrequent and of relatively little interest to students of psychopathology' (p.276).

A number of factors contributed to the comparative lack of interest in Alzheimer's disease at this time. The first was general loss of influence of Kraepelin's account of the organic basis of mental illness. This loss of influence is most clearly seen in explanations of schizophrenia. It would appear that the reclusive Kraepelin had lost academic ground in the years preceding the First World War.

> Before his settling in Munich, Kraepelin had had long years of collaboration with Gustav Aschaffenburg who contributed papers to the 'Psychologische Arbeiten'. After Kraepelin's arrival in Munich his relationship with Aschaffenburg seemed to have cooled. Never discussing personal matters, Kraepelin has not mentioned the relationship between himself and Aschaffenburg. However, when Aschaffenburg's twelve volume Handbuch der Psychiatry appeared, Kraepelin's name appeared neither as a collaborator nor as a member of the editorial board. However, there is an entire volume devoted to Dementia Praecox. But this volume was written by Eugene Bleuler who bent the concept of Dementia Praecox to that of Schizophrenia. (Harms 1971, pp.xvi–xvii)

As we have described above, Kraepelin's account of mental illness stressed the role of organic changes occurring within the brain and largely excluded personal and social factors from consideration. This contrasted with Bleuler's (1950 [first published 1911]) approach, which drew on writings that linked mental illness to unconscious processes, such as those of Freud.

Second, the evidence that senile dementia represented a separate condition from ageing rather than just an accelerated form of it was inconclusive in this period. The Newcastle group (Blessed, Roth and Tomlinson) had shown a correlation between memory difficulties and intensity of plaque formation (Roth *et al.* 1966; 1967; Blessed *et al.* 1968; Tomlinson *et al.* 1968; 1970). However, the pathological changes associated with Alzheimer's disease (neurofibrillary plaques and tangles) were also found in the brains of individuals who had aged normally. Thus 'there was good evidence that, at a histological level, the difference between patients with AD and intellectually normal older adults is quantitative rather than qualitative' (Hart and Semple 1994, p.44). So, even with the correlational evidence from the Newcastle group that was available by the seventies, Alzheimer's disease and dementia more generally were still not clearly established as diseases that could be distinguished from ageing.

Moreover, dementia itself was relatively rare for much of this period. Pre-senile dementia (dementia before the age of sixty) is statistically infrequent and, because it was thought to be untreatable, rarely came to medical attention. Dementia amongst the over-65s was also little researched, for a variety of reasons. Not only was the life expectancy comparatively short by today's standards, but many older people with dementia would die relatively early in the course of the illness from diseases which could not be treated before the advent of antibiotics.

By the middle of the 1970s a number of factors had combined to raise the profile of age-related illnesses. Probably the most important of these influences was the increase in life expectancy in most Western countries. By the 1960s average life expectancy in the United Kingdom had risen to 68 for men and 74 for women, compared to 1930 figures of 59 and 63 respectively. That this demographic change was represented as a potential threat to society is illustrated by the report of the Health Advisory Service published in 1982 entitled *The Rising Tide: Developing Services for Mental Illness in Old Age* – a remarkable juxtaposition of a modest aim with highly-charged imagery. The suggestion is that an ageing population with high rates of illness will create a demand that cannot be met or financed. This fear of an overstretched health service collapsing under the strain of the needs of the elderly was not restricted to the United Kingdom. For example, a paper from Australia is titled 'The coming epidemic of dementia' (Henderson 1983). Yet the imminent collapse did not have a great deal of reality to it.

> Because the problem of dementia is often reported in exaggerated tones,
> it is worth emphasising that only 1.1 percent of the population of
> Scotland in 1994 had dementia, and 6.9 percent of those aged 65 and
> over – substantial figures but hardly likely to bring about the collapse of
> civilisation as we know it. (Gordon and Spicker 1997, p.45)

It is certainly the case that there were demographic changes. What was
remarkable was the fear and panic that these changes caused. These fears
could be utilised by those wishing to gain more funding for research into
dementia, especially if the public believed that increased funding would
bring about a cure. This process happened in Britain to a limited extent, but
was much more important (and better documented) in the United States.

What was remarkable, then, was that these changes were framed in such
catastrophic and dramatic terms. Alongside these demographic changes was
another change – a re-framing of dementia, and in particular Alzheimer's
disease. This involved the transformation of Alzheimer's disease from the
most common form of a rare illness (pre-senile dementia) into the fourth or
fifth leading cause of death in the United States in little more than 12 years
(Fox 1989, p.58). The mechanism by which this repositioning of Alzheimer's
disease occurred has a number of parallels with the original creation of
Alzheimer's disease by Kraepelin in 1910. In particular, there was a strategic
decision to broaden the conceptual boundaries of Alzheimer's disease. In this
enlarged state, it was then incorporated within a more general psychiatric
framework which once again emphasised organic rather than psychosocial
factors.

The first person to suggest such a repositioning of Alzheimer's disease
was a neurologist, Robert Katzman. In 1974 he prepared a paper with
Toksoz Karasu to present at the Houston Neurological Symposium (1975).

> The first suggestion, which Katzman estimated from existing
> epidemiological data, was that 'senile dementia' was the 4th leading
> cause of death in the United States. The second suggestion, based on the
> work or Ralph Terry and other researchers, was that senile dementia and
> Alzheimer's disease were the same entity: 'We should like to make the
> suggestion, simplistic as it may be, that we should drop the term "senile
> dementia" and include these cases under the diagnosis of Alzheimer's
> Disease.' (Katzman and Karasu 1975, p.106) (Fox 1989, p.71)

What Katzman and others were proposing was that there was evidence to
suggest that senile and pre-senile dementia were one and the same thing, and
that therefore the distinction between the two should be dropped and the

resulting concept termed Alzheimer's disease. Yet even were there evidence that Alzheimer's disease and senile dementia were synonymous, *the logic would be to drop the less frequent, less inclusive condition.* To use an economic analogy, the adoption of Alzheimer's disease as the descriptive category was the equivalent of a local corner shop taking over a national supermarket chain.

As we can see from the quotation from Fox above (*see also* Harding and Palfrey 1997), Katzman used two arguments to justify this re-framing.

Morbidity

It is hard to substantiate the claim that dementia is the sole cause of death in the way that Katzman suggested. For instance, Gilleard (1984) concluded: 'The expected survival of elderly individuals developing dementia does not greatly differ from that of elderly individuals not developing dementia, unless the onset of mental decline occurs before the age of 75' (quoted in Ineichen 1987, p.198). As Kitwood has pointed out, there is a difference between a person dying *with* dementia and a person dying *from* dementia (1997b).

Yet, suggesting that dementia was such a high cause of death was an important part of the repositioning of dementia and the re-creation of Alzheimer's disease. Implicit within Katzman's argument was the belief that biomedical research into senile dementia had been under-resourced and that establishing it as an illness with a high mortality rate rather than as an aspect of ageing would aid attempts to attract greater funding. As Fox points out, this argument did indeed have two benefits in terms of potential funding. It 'increased' the frequency of Alzheimer's in the population manyfold, and equally crucially, it medicalised old age. You could do little about getting older, but you could argue for financial help to study a disease, especially if by framing this disease as originating in organic changes within the brain you could argue that biomedical research would produce a cure. The re-creation of Alzheimer's disease can be seen as the creation of mental illnesses through the medicalisation of old age (Adelman 1995; Estes and Binney 1989). Perhaps behind both was the fear of dying and the hope that it could be postponed indefinitely (Gubrium 1986).

It is clear that re-labelling senile dementia as Alzheimer's disease was indeed extremely successful. The budget allocated to research on Alzheimer's within the main federal funding body grew from 0.8 million dollars in 1976 (4.4 per cent of its budget) to 80 million dollars in 1989 (35.9 per cent of its budget) (Fox 1989).

The continuum model

The second argument that Katzman used to justify the repositioning of senile dementia arose from research that suggested that there was one disease entity and not two. There are clear parallels with the arguments surrounding Kraepelin's creation of Alzheimer's disease that we have detailed above. First of all, just as Kraepelin and Alzheimer had used the technology of histology to substantiate their claims, so Terry's (1963) innovation was to use electron microscopy to study brain diseases.

Second, in an ironic twist, what Katzman and others proposed was that far from being a disease entity separate from other forms of dementia, as Kraepelin had argued, Alzheimer's disease in younger adults was identical to the dementia found in older adults. In essence this marked a return to the claim that Alzheimer himself had made about Frau Auguste D – that she represented an atypical form of dementia only in the sense that she was in her mid-fifties at the time of her death.

The final parallel between this re-creation of Alzheimer's disease and the rhetorical claims of Kraepelin lies in the establishment of Alzheimer's disease within a wider psychiatric framework – in this case the Diagnostic and Statistical Manual of Mental Disorders (DSM) produced by the American Psychiatric Association. Relatively little attention had been paid to the first two editions of this diagnostic manual. However, at the point at which the third revision was being produced in the late 1970s, a series of arguments were raging over the diagnostic categories that should be included within it, such as for example whether or not homosexuality was a psychiatric disorder (Bayer 1981).

Just as Kraepelin had produced his textbooks as a means of establishing his (organic) representations of mental illness as the dominant frame, so the DSM series can be seen as an attempt to establish a particular form of psychiatric representation as the dominant mode of knowing. Just as Kraepelin had to compete with the alternative accounts presented by Bleuler, so, if American psychiatry in the 1970s was to keep control of the mental health system, it had to be the authority that specified what mental illnesses were and what criteria had to be fulfilled for a diagnosis of a particular illness to be established. Not only would such an enterprise downgrade paramedical professions such as clinical psychology and social work, who did not have the power to establish such diagnoses, it would also take power and prestige away from psychoanalysts, who found little utility in such a diagnostic framework (Kirk and Kutchins 1992).

Thus, for both Kraepelin and the authors of DSM III, there were major issues concerning professional power within both the psychiatric system and the wider health care environment (Kirk and Kutchins 1992). The publication of DSM III was framed as the arrival of scientific psychiatry (e.g. Klerman 1984; Maxmen 1985). This represented an attempt to establish psychiatry as the science of mental illnesses or specified diseases rather than the art of helping people in distress or of understanding failures to communicate and dysfunctional systems.

Within five years of Katzman and Karasin's Houston paper (1975), DSM III was able to pronounce that 'Primary Degenerative Dementia of the Alzheimer type is the most common dementia' (American Psychiatric Association 1980, p.110). But establishing 'Alzheimer's disease' as the major type of dementia did not answer the questions that were being asked about the nature of dementia at the end of the nineteenth century. The enshrining of Alzheimer's in DSM III and the whole codification process implied and applied in DSM III was scientific advance by proclamation. Indeed, it was actually a retrogression in terms of scientific endeavour compared to the work of the Munich department. Whereas Kraepelin had been concerned to divide dementia into separate sub-groupings, DSM III expanded vastly what was at that point a relatively minor disease category.

The nomenclature was made looser and more confused with the emergence of carer pressure groups. In both Britain and America organisations used the name 'Alzheimer's Disease Society' but were concerned with all forms of dementia. Thus by the mid 1980s 'Alzheimer's Disease' had three meanings: (1) pre-senile dementia with a particular histological configuration; (2) senile dementia with the same configuration; and (3) all forms of dementia.

Postscript

We do not know a great deal about Alois Alzheimer. He seems to have been at his happiest when looking down a microscope and trying to utilise the most up-to-date staining techniques to elucidate what he saw. He married at 30 but by 1901, at the age of 37, he was widowed with three young children. He has been described as never overcoming his wife's early death, instead throwing himself into his histological studies (Hoff 1991, p.31).

> From 1903 to 1912, his years in Munich, Alzheimer became a well loved figure to students from all over the world. He would spend hours with each one, explaining things as they shared a microscope, always with a

cigar that would be put down as he commenced his explanations and it is said that at the end of the day there would always be a cigar stump at every student's bench by the microscope. (Hoff 1991, p.33)

In 1912, two years after Kraepelin had created the disease that bore his name, Alzheimer accepted the post of Professor of Psychiatry at Breslau, far to the east of the Hapsburg Empire and the academic centres of Germany. Kraepelin had urged him to stay in Munich (Burns *et al.* 1995, p.1). We may speculate whether one of his reasons for leaving the security and prestige of Kraepelin's department was that he knew that he had to stop living out Kraepelin's claim that he, Alzheimer, had found a new disease; a claim which, having little substance, had to be shored up with papers by members of his team exaggerating the number of exemplars by sharing the same histological specimens. And if he knew that Kraepelin had been over-optimistic in his conclusion, he would have had even less enthusiasm for the re-creation of Alzheimer's disease sixty years later as an explanation for the mental infirmities of old age.

Alzheimer was never to return from the east. On the train journey to Breslau he fell ill with tonsillitis, later complicated with nephritis and arthritis (Burns *et al.* 1995, p.1). He died aged 51, the age of Frau Auguste D when she was admitted.

Summary of main points

- In 1910, Kraepelin used Alzheimer's name to create a disease to help keep his institution in the forefront of organic psychiatry.
- In the 1980s, Alzheimer's name was used to gain funding for biomedical research into brain disorders. The re-creation of Alzheimer's disease may have facilitated an explosion in funding for biomedical research, but it has also served to place people with Alzheimer's disease within a constricting explanatory framework in which they tend to be perceived as diseased brains rather than as social beings with active mental lives. The creation and re-creation of Alzheimer's disease, with its emphasis upon organic changes occurring within the brain, has involved a loss of explanatory accounts just as one particular account (the organic) has become more detailed.
- The greatest need of people with dementia is to be treated with respect, as paid-up members of the human race rather than as diseased brains (Kitwood 1997b). Deciding that Alzheimer's disease

'exists' because it is in the DSM does not clarify either what happens to people when they lose their skills and abilities or the dialectical relationship that exists between the individual and their social context. (Kitwood 1988; 1990a; Kitwood and Bredin 1992; Harding and Palfry 1997)

- In this chapter we have examined the concept of dementia in its historical context. We have discussed possible alternative explanations of Frau Auguste D's condition. We hope we have also shown how 'the great man/inevitability of scientific progress' frame does not fit well with the actual history of Alzheimer's disease. In the next chapter we look at contemporary explanations of dementia.

The Present Formulation
of Dementia

In this chapter we outline the main elements of the contemporary biomedical model of dementia. The main aims of this chapter are:

- to explore the ways in which explanations of behaviour that is different or 'odd' are socially determined
- to set out the various definitions of dementia, its main symptoms and its causes
- to outline the major illnesses (Alzheimer's, multi-infarct and Lewy-body) and some of the less common conditions
- and finally, to look at contemporary ideas about the genetics of dementia, its frequency and its risk factors.

Some people's behaviours are so odd and different that it seems self-evident that *they* are different. The things that they do and the way that they speak are apparently so illogical that they are outside the range of experience of most members of their society. Such aberrant behaviour requires an explanation. Those who display it could be perceived as being 'possessed of the devil' like medieval witches, who were probably reclusive, eccentric ladies; or they could be seen as 'bad', as were the starving people who were hung for steeling sheep as recently as 150 years ago. These are 'negative' explanations in the sense that they have quite painful consequences for those whose behaviour is so explained and made sense of. Such behaviour is not always explained negatively, however. In the Inuit culture, people with epilepsy are more likely to become shamans (Lewis 1971).

To illustrate a range of possible frameworks, Box 2.1 outlines briefly a variety of perspectives from the social sciences. Some, such as griefwork and attachment theory, we will elaborate on later in the text, but the main purpose of Box 2.1 is to show the rich variety of approaches that could illuminate our understanding of dementia.

Box 2.1 Possible explanations of dementia

The organic disease model has achieved paradigmatic status (Kuhn 1962). That is to say, there is near-uniform agreement that within this model lies the explanation of dementia. This monolithic approach has quite severe consequences in terms of excluding other perspectives. In our introduction, we mentioned the sociological and the psychological perspectives. But we can be more exact as to the loss of potential useful alternatives. Whilst these models might seem abstract, almost all combat the therapeutic nihilism of the organic model. If they *could* help and benefit people with dementia then the validity of the organic model would need to be questioned.

1. *Political/historical*: How does thinking about dementia reflect the needs of the country at a given time?

2. *Sociological/professional*: Marshall (1996) talks of the various professions each fiercely guarding their own territory and boundaries. How does this tribalism explain developments in the field of dementia? One way in which it certainly does can be seen in the development and increased importance of psychiatric classification. The development of the DSM series (1980; 1994) is clearly documented as a fight between two tribes within psychiatry (Kirk and Kutchins 1992).

3. *Dementia as a disability*: There is a large literature on disability, mainly in relation to physical handicaps. The disability model has the merit of specifying what is actually missing/damaged, unlike a model of a disease that eats into all abilities and personhood. Therefore, a disability model could specify more exactly how a person with dementia could be helped and how their environment could be more user-friendly.

4. *Dementia as deviance* : To what extent is it useful to see dementia not as a disease but as a ragbag of behaviour that upsets the unwritten 'laws' of social behaviour? (Scheff 1966). If no one was worried about these infringements would they worry about dementia?

5. *Dementia as brain damage (1)*: Road Traffic Accident patients receive much more substantial and detailed assessments than people with dementia. They also get detailed treatment programmes, which almost never happens with people who are diagnosed as having dementia.

6. *Dementia as brain damage (2)*: If dementia results in the loss of major functional skills then the behaviour of people with dementia might well have similarities with people who have severe learning difficulties. An obvious overlap, for

---

Box 2.1 continued

example is the work of Wolfensberger on normalisation[1] (1972; 1992) and Kitwood on malignant social psychology[2] (1990a). Another, as Marshall (1996) points out, is that advocacy has been found to be very useful in the field of learning difficulty but has not been introduced with older clients. So, potentially useful techniques have been confined to specialisms within psychological work for separate client groups.

7. *Dementia as a major functional illness*: The odd thing about people with dementia is that only about a third of them are classified as depressed, though figures vary widely. So, we have an incongruity of affect – we might expect them to be very depressed, if not suicidal, but they are not. Could dementia be the result of descending, in old age, into existential meaninglessness?

8. *Dementia as a psychosis*: In schizophrenia, we get symptoms such as incongruity of affect, flatness of affect and thought disorder. How alike or dissimilar are these to similar behaviours found in dementia?

   There is some overlap in the next few framings, all of which relate to the psychological.

9. *Dementia as a subjective state*: To believe you are losing your mind must be terrifying and in some of the autobiographical accounts, most noticeably the Reverend Davis' *My Journey into Alzheimer's Disease* (1989) and also in some carer accounts (Ignatieff's *Scar Tissue* (1993) and Heywood's *Caring for Maria* (1994), this is all too obvious.

   But we have no models of people in this state of 'fear and trembling' (Kierkegaard 1954, originally published 1843).

10. *Dementia as regression*: To what extent can dementia be seen as a loss of security which is so severe that the person feels vulnerable as they did when, as a very young infant, their parent(s) provided their only security? Attachment theory might be a very useful explanatory tool (Miesen 1992; 1993) see Chapter 8.

11. *Dementia as loss*: To what extent can we see the person with dementia as grieving for their lost skills, lost relationships and a lost lifestyle? In this sense dementia can be seen as unsuccessful griefwork (Worden 1991).

12. *Dementia as trauma*: To what extent is it useful to conceptualise that when a person becomes convinced that they have dementia they are overwhelmed by this realisation? If this is so then we could consider them to be in a state of post-traumatic shock (Hunt, Marshall and Rowlings 1997).

---

1   Normalisation – the provision of valued social roles

2   Malignant Social Psychology – those aspects of the social world which impair the personhood of the person with dementia

We cannot blame the organic model completely for the unpopularity of alternative models; to this we would have to add the fragmentation of academic disciplines and ever-increasing specialisation within areas and departments. But certainly, the assumption of the correctness of only one model has further hindered cross-frame work.

In this century, the 'illness' model has been used to explain an increasing range of behaviours that people in our society find difficult to comprehend or deal with. One of the areas of behaviour that people find difficult is getting old and dying. We are frightened of ceasing to exist. Ceasing to exist whilst still alive is even more painful to contemplate. Yet it is the term 'living death' that Woods (1989) used so evocatively to describe dementia. Our society puts great emphasis on thinking quickly and effectively. People who cannot do this frighten us, perhaps because one day we might be like them. So people with dementia certainly do things that we find hard to handle.

In our society, one of the major ways of understanding 'odd' behaviours is to say that the person displaying them is 'ill'. We can juxtapose our commonsensical behaviour with their illness, in this case a type of mental illness. Put like this, it might seem that we have plenty of choice in deciding how we will understand 'odd', unusual or frightening behaviour. But this is only true to a limited extent. Because we are 'inside' our society certain ways of explaining events seem 'natural'. As a consequence, most people probably think that people with dementia act in such a bizarre way that what they do and say makes no sense at all. It seems to be just a matter of 'common sense' to describe people who act in such a bizarre way as 'mad' or 'insane'. It is not surprising, then, that we, as a society, have developed a way of thinking about dementia as an illness – a psychiatric illness.

It seems only natural, therefore, that people with dementia should be treated by psychiatrists and psychiatric nurses in the same way in which people who are physically ill are treated by ordinary doctors and nurses. If we are to understand what dementia 'is' and what it is like to 'have' dementia, then a sensible starting place is to understand the main explanations of and treatments for dementia, and to look at the medical or psychiatric way of thinking about illness.

Diagnosis and classification

By and large, the medical way of thinking about people is that they are either well or ill – one or the other. The psychiatrist is concerned with looking for particular symptoms and groups of symptoms which will allow him or her to make a diagnosis, just as any doctor would look for particular symptoms to allow him or her to say whether, for instance, a stomach pain is a sign of indigestion, a hernia or appendicitis. The psychiatrist will be concerned with how long these symptoms have existed and will make a number of judgements about the patient – about the reality of his or her beliefs, for instance, and about how much these symptoms affect his or her life and the lives of those around him or her. They will aim to get all the relevant information needed in order for a diagnosis to be made.

A central issue, then, is diagnosis. If the doctor sees certain symptoms, then a specific diagnosis is given, and from this a specific treatment follows. If this treatment does not work, then other – perhaps more intense – treatments are called for or a new diagnosis needs to be made.

There are good, practical reasons for taking this classificatory approach. If every person is thought of as unique – if there is no way of classifying people at all – then no case law could be built up. In effect, we would be unable to see the wood for the trees. It is only by classifying into categories, then classifying further into subtypes and then investigating each subtype that medical knowledge has been able to progress systematically to a point at which many illnesses can be cured.

Essentially, a diagnosis identifies an individual as a member of a specific group of patients. For each group a number of different treatment options are available. In contemporary psychiatry, these tend to be pharmacological – the doctor prescribes a particular medication. This is not surprising, really, given the apparent success of medicine in combating physical disease and illness. Recently we have had some evidence of the usefulness of such an approach – the first drug for improving a person's ability to remember, known as Aricept, was licensed for use in the UK in 1997. This drug, it is claimed, provides the first opportunity to chemically enhance the memories of people with dementia. We will discuss Aricept in more detail later on.

This description of the psychiatric model is inevitably rather simplistic, and so far we have ignored the fact that, no matter what criteria are developed, the process whereby a diagnosis is reached is inevitably a subjective one carried out by fallible human beings. Moreover, it is these fallible human beings who have to decide what is and is not an illness. Over time these decisions about illness and symptoms have changed, so that we now recognise as illnesses sets of behaviours that even 20 years ago would have been disregarded or seen as evidence of moral weakness. One example of this is the acknowledgement that people who have been involved in a traumatic event may later suffer from post-traumatic stress disorder. Not so many years ago these forms of reaction were seen as the result of personal psychological instability rather than a 'genuine' illness arising from trauma. Similarly, the converse also holds, and often what used to be seen as illnesses are no longer viewed as such – most people in society do not now regard homosexuality as an illness, for example. Less dramatically, the meaning attached to particular diagnoses also changes, as we have seen was the case with Alzheimer's disease.

Psychiatric systems of classification

At present two important systems of classifying psychiatric illnesses exist. The World Health Organisation sponsored the development, in 1948, of the International Classification of Diseases (ICD); in the US a slightly different system emerged known as the American Psychiatric Association Diagnostic and Statistical Manual (DSM). Both of these systems have gone through many variations, with some illnesses being abandoned, others brought into being and most altered, some radically. The latest versions are ICD 10 (WHO 1992) and DSM IV (APA 1994).

The symptoms listed in order to create a diagnosis still differ slightly from system to system. Therefore, actual diagnostic practices vary according to the system of diagnoses being used and the time at which the diagnosis is made. For instance, as we have shown in Chapter 1 in the 1970s, before the third edition of the DSM, Alzheimer's disease was defined as a pre-senile dementia: an illness which only affected younger people. Later editions of the DSM have defined Alzheimer's disease in a much broader and therefore more inclusive way (American Psychiatric Association 1980; 1994). The reasons for this shift are complicated but have much to do with the need to define dementia in a way that will be attractive to potential sources of research money. After all, you can claim to be able to find the cure for a disease in a way that you cannot for old age or senility.

Examples of psychiatric diagnosis from DSM IV are given in Box 2.2.

Box 2.2 Some examples of 'psychiatric illness'

Schizophrenic disorders: unrelated conversation; delusions; hallucinations; loss of contact with world and with other people.

Affective disorders: depression, mania.

Anxiety disorders: phobias, panic attacks, generalised anxiety, obsessive-compulsive disorders.

Personality disorders include: *Schizoid personality*: aloof, few friends, indifferent to praise or criticism; *Narcissistic personality*: overblown sense of self-importance, fantasies about great success, requires constant attention; *Anti-social personality*: surfaces before age 15, irresponsible, doesn't plan ahead, indifferent to the law.

The diagnosis of dementia

The term 'dementia' is used to refer to two related concepts: to a syndrome that comprises a broad pattern of clinical symptoms; and to a number of specific although potentially related diseases (Lishman 1987). Thus the term 'Alzheimer's disease' can 1) mean a specific illness, the parameters of which have changed over the years, or 2) be an all-encompassing term for a broad range of conditions (the Alzheimer's Disease Society, for instance, is really for anyone caring for a relative who has a dementing illness).

The syndrome of dementia

The International Classification of Diseases produced by the World Health Organisation (1992) offers the following definition:

> Dementia is a syndrome due to disease of the brain, usually of a chronic or progressive nature, in which there is a disturbance of multiple higher cortical functions, including memory, thinking, orientation, comprehension, calculation, learning capacity, language, and judgement. Consciousness is not clouded. Impairments of cognitive function are commonly accompanied, and occasionally preceded, by deterioration in emotional control, social behaviour or motivation.
>
> The primary requirement for diagnosis is evidence of decline in both memory and thinking which is sufficient to impair personal activities of daily living ... The above symptoms and impairments should have been evident for at least six months for a confident diagnosis of dementia to be made.

The American Psychiatric Association DSM IV (1994) offers a slightly different definition, which does not require evidence of chronicity or progression. This has five separate elements:

A. Impairment in short and long-term memory.
B. At least one of:
    i)   impairment in abstract thinking
    ii)   impaired judgement
    iii) other disturbances of higher cortical functioning
    iv)   personality change.
C. That the deficit in A and B significantly interferes with work or social activities.
D. That these deficits should not be caused by delirium.
E. Either there is evidence from the person's history or a physical examination to show that the deficits are produced by a dementia or these problems cannot be accounted for by any other condition.

Dementia is a diagnosis by exclusion – it is what you have left when you have excluded all other sources of confused behaviour. This is an important point that we will return to later in the chapter; essentially it means that a diagnosis of dementia is often reached when the person doing the diagnosis cannot find any other explanation for the problems the person is experiencing.

It is because of the diagnostic approach that we know that some forms of confusion can be treated and that some forms of confusion are reversible. For example, if an elderly person contracts an infection of the bladder this can often cause them to become confused and unsure of themselves. This is called a Urinary Tract Infection (UTI) and can usually be cured simply by the prescription of a dose of antibiotics.

Once we have excluded all other possible causes of confusion and arrived at a diagnosis of dementia of one form or another, then it is still the case that we cannot predict with any certainty what symptoms will occur or how the illness will progress, other than that the person with dementia will deteriorate.

The extent to which people with dementia are affected by their illness varies, ranging from forgetfulness and other eccentricities that most people would regard as socially tolerable through to the loss of effective psychological functioning. These variations are not just due to the fact that the illness is progressive and sufferers can be expected to deteriorate. It is also because there are huge variations in how people are affected by the course of dementia, from one form of the illness to another and from person to person.

On a clinical basis, some of the most common changes that may indicate that a person is suffering from a dementing illness include:

- a deteriorating memory, especially for recent events
- difficulty in learning new information
- difficulty in handling complex tasks
- an impairment of the ability to reason and to think in more abstract terms
- problems in using language to express themselves
- changes in behaviour, perhaps including wandering and restlessness, difficulty in holding a sensible conversation, being unusually rude, giving up previous interests and hobbies, and being uninterested in papers or TV
- emotional changes such as emotional blunting, self-neglect, and a general lack of initiative.

There have been a number of attempts to identify different *phases* or *stages* of the dementing illness. DSM IV follows a common trend of viewing dementia as progressing from a first, early stage of forgetfulness to a middle, confusional phase when cognitive deficits are readily apparent to an observer. Finally there is the late 'dementia' phase, by which point the individual is no longer capable of an independent life. Similarly, in terms of *severity*, dementia is often classified as being mild, moderate or severe. Thus:

- *Mild dementia* results in difficulties with work or social activities, but the person with dementia is still able to live independently, maintain adequate personal hygiene and exercise a reasonable amount of judgement in their life.
- As the dementia progresses to a *moderate* level of impairment, independent living becomes more hazardous.
- *Severe dementia* refers to a state in which the activities of daily living are so impaired that continuous support is required; for example, people with a severe level of dementia are seen as unable to maintain even minimal hygiene and are often mute or largely incoherent.

Other illnesses which can be mistaken for dementia

Amongst the most common and reversible illnesses that can be mistaken for dementia are depression and delirium. These are examples of what many doctors refer to as pseudodementias: that is to say, conditions that appear to be similar to a dementing illness but which are in fact relatively easily treated and alleviated.

Delirium can be mistaken for dementia, and tends to be characterised by a sudden onset of a similar set of symptoms, but also tends to include hallucinations, misinterpretation of events and a clouding of consciousness. Delirium can be excluded by a careful checking of the individual's history and in particular their use of medication and alcohol.

Table 2.1 Distinguishing dementia from confusion

Confusion can result from a number of causes and is much more common than dementia. Therefore:

1. All possible reasons for confused behaviour should be investigated as soon as possible.

2. Dementia should only be considered when other causes have definitely been ruled out.

Possible reasons for confusion:

1. Residents having insufficient information, e.g. not knowing where the toilet or dining room is.

2. Staff having insufficient information about residents. Are they hard of hearing? Can they see properly?

3. Acute confusional states. These can be caused by infections (especially urinary tract infections and chest infections), congestive heart failure, hypothyroidism, diabetes, b12 deficiency, concussion and some drugs.

4. Chronic confusional states. These can occur in terminal cancer, kidney failure and liver failure as toxic matter builds up in the body.

5. Anxiety.

6. Speech difficulties.

7. Resentment and anger.

8. Grief.

9. Depression.

Depression is thought to be probably the most frequent cause of misdiagnoses of dementia. When a person suffers from a depression rather than a dementia there tends to be a history of depression either in their own life or within their family, and often an external cause (a life event such as a bereavement or other loss). People who are depressed are more likely to experience a range of what doctors call somatic problems such as waking early, to be more depressed in the morning than later on and to move and react more slowly. They also tend to make more self-deprecating remarks and have a lower opinion of their own abilities than is actually the case. Often the best test of whether a person has depression rather than dementia is to start them on a course of anti-depressant medication and see if they improve.

The relationship between depression and dementia is a complex one, however. For instance, a person may well have both dementia and depression, thus making diagnosis very difficult. We will return to this complex relationship between depression and dementia in Chapter 9.

Specific sub-diagnostic types of dementia

Three main subtypes of dementia are distinguished: a) Dementia of the Alzheimer's type (DAT); b) Vascular dementia, also known as multi-infarct dementia (MID); and c) Lewy-body dementia (LBD). These illnesses are generally characterised as having the following characteristics:

Dementia of the Alzheimer's type (DAT)

This form of dementia is perhaps the most common, with studies suggesting that up to two-thirds of all dementias fall within this category. DAT is thought to result from neurological changes (amyloid plaques and neurofibrillary tangles) within the brain.

DAT is a global impairment affecting almost all of a person's intellectual abilities. Although the illness typically involves a gradual and progressive decline, nevertheless individuals can still have plateaus of up to a year during which there is either no or relatively little loss of abilities. The earliest changes tend to be seen in the sufferer's language; they may have problems naming even common objects such as a watch. Visual abilities such as recognising people, finding one's way around or drawing are also affected, while socially appropriate behaviour (including making professional judgements of complex situations) can also begin to deteriorate.

Vascular dementia or multi-infarct dementia (MID)

Vascular dementias account for perhaps 10–20 per cent of all diagnosed forms of dementia. A series of small strokes or infarcts occur, with a typically abrupt onset. There is usually said to be a sudden deterioration in the patient's condition after each stroke, followed by some recovery. Consequently the typical pattern is thought to be one of a patchy and stepwise decline in abilities, with some areas affected more than others. Vascular dementias will be accompanied by other signs of the infarcts such as physical weakness and, perhaps, temporary loss of movement in some parts of the body.

Lewy-body dementia (LBD)

This subtype has only been identified relatively recently, but some studies suggest that LBD accounts for 7–30 per cent of diagnosed dementia patients. The illness gains its name from the presence of so-called 'Lewy bodies', which are distinctive tiny spherical structures found in the nerve cells of the brain, especially within the frontal, temporal and parietal lobes. It is thought these structures may contribute to the death of brain cells.

Clinically, LBD is often mild at the outset and can be extremely variable from day to day. Patients with LBD experience the early appearance of what are known as extrapyramidal symptoms (difficulty in initiating movements and physical rigidity) which do not respond to medication with dopamine (unlike most symptoms of this sort, for instance those due to Parkinson's disease). The person with LBD may also be extremely confused, experiencing delusions and hallucinations. In many ways the duration of the illness and the sort of cognitive impairments found in people with LBD are similar to those of people with Alzheimer's disease. Because of the similarities with both DAT and Parkinson's disease, there is disagreement over whether LBD is a distinct illness, a variant of DAT or a part of Parkinson's disease.

Less common forms of dementing illness

Frontal lobe dementia (FLD)

Frontal lobe dementia is much less common than Alzheimer's disease, and is thought to account for less than 10 per cent of all dementias. Many different illnesses are associated with the degeneration of the frontal lobes, of which one of the most well known is Pick's disease (named after Arnold Pick, who first described the disease at the turn of the century). Pick's disease is most common among people aged under 65. People who develop Pick's disease will live, on average, for about seven years.

As the term 'Frontal lobe dementia' suggests, the primary features seen early in the disease are those controlled by the frontal lobes of the brain; they include apathy, outbursts of aggression, disinhibited or inappropriate social behaviour, inattention, neglect of personal hygiene, loss of insight and perseveration (the sufferer has difficulty in moving from one thought or action to another and repeats him- or herself over and over again). Sufferers often tend to become less inhibited about expressing themselves, and may become obsessional or seem to lose interest in life. Occasionally Pick's disease will affect the temporal lobes more than the frontal lobes. In these cases the early symptoms are more likely to involve memory loss and difficulty in recognising ordinary objects. There may also be a change in eating habits, with the sufferer wanting to eat sweet things or eat far too much.

Post-traumatic dementia (Dementia pugilistica)

Closed head trauma is the most common head injury that can later produce dementia, being present in about 2 per cent of all cases of dementia. It is clear that repeated blows to the head can cause dementia, although a very severe single head injury can also do so. Boxing is one of the professions most at risk of developing post-traumatic dementia (it has been estimated that Mohammed Ali received over 25,000 blows to his head during his career). In boxers with dementia pugilistica, neurofibrillary tangles are found in all areas of the neocortex. However, in contrast to DAT, there are relatively few plaques and amyloid deposits.

Post-traumatic dementia shows a combination of dementia and extrapyramidal signs. In addition to a variety of behavioural and cognitive impairments, especially those caused by damage to the frontal areas of the brain, specific symptoms can occur. These include aphasia (forgetting the names of objects), amnesia, inattention, slowed thinking, confusion and memory loss. The deficits from post-traumatic dementia depend upon the severity of the head injury and the locations of the brain damage. The recovery time, if complete, is months for minor head injuries, and from years to never for severe head injuries.

Creutzfeldt-Jakob disease (CJD)

This disease is a human form of transmissible dementia. It is known as scrapie in sheep and bovine spongiform encephalopathy (BSE) in cows. Like all transmissible dementias, CJD has a long latency period but progresses very rapidly once symptoms appear. Initially there may be behavioural disturbances, spasmodic movements, unsteadiness and tremors. There is no treatment as yet, and death usually occurs within months rather than years. Despite recent publicity, CJD is still an extremely rare disease. A number of possible causes have been identified, including genetic predisposition and environmental triggers. CJD has also been transmitted accidentally through surgical procedures and the use of growth hormone treatment using infected human pituitary glands.

There is controversy over whether a new variant of CJD, particularly affecting young people, has arisen as a result of the BSE epidemic in Britain. BSE is thought to be caused by a rare infectious agent which is quite different from either a bacteria or a virus. Researchers have termed this agent a 'prion' (hence these are sometimes called 'prion diseases') which is a form of protein. Unlike other infectious agents, the prion does not replicate itself through DNA, which makes it extremely difficult to destroy. In the case of BSE the prion appears to have been passed from sheep to cows through the use of infected brain material in feed. Subsequently this has given rise to concern that the agent could be transmitted to humans through eating beef or beef products containing infected nervous tissue. Accordingly, a range of preventive measures have been taken.

Parkinson's disease

This neurological disorder is caused by the gradual loss of a chemical messenger called dopamine from the part of the brain which controls movement. Symptoms vary, but can include tremor, stiffness, slowness and difficulty in starting to move. It is thought that 15 to 20 per cent of people with Parkinson's disease also have dementia.

Huntington's disease

This is an inherited disease in which a faulty gene on chromosome 4 leads to degeneration of nerve cells in certain parts of the brain. The disease usually appears between the ages of 30 and 50, with early symptoms including forgetfulness, clumsiness, depression and irrational behaviour. Dementia occurs in the majority of cases. There is no treatment yet available to halt the progress of the disease, but some of the symptoms can be relieved by drugs.

Box 2.3 Possible biological and genetic bases for Alzheimer's disease: current formulations

One of the major areas of neurological and medical research has focused on identifying those environmental and genetic risk factors which predispose an individual to develop Alzheimer's disease and other dementias. A number of predisposing and preventive factors have been identified, although the role of hereditary factors has perhaps attracted the most attention. Several genes have been identified that appear to affect the probability that an individual will be affected by DAT. These genes run in families and are usually associated with an early onset (prior to 60 years of age) and an unusually high incidence of Alzheimer's disease within the family.

Of more general interest, however, has been the recent discovery of the importance of the apolipoprotein E gene (E4) on chromosome 19 in the pathogenesis of late-onset Alzheimer's disease (Golden 1995; Stephens 1995). Each person has two copies of the Apo E gene, and there are three different possible forms (alleles) of it (Apo E2, 3 and 4). Thus an individual could have any one of six possible combinations of this particular gene (Apo E2/2, 3/3, 4/4, 2/3, 3/4 and 2/4).

The exact combination of Apo E that an individual has seems to affect their susceptibility to Alzheimer's disease. Although Alzheimer's disease can occur with all genotypes, the inheritance of either one or two Apo E4 alleles is associated with earlier onset of the disease. The relative risk of developing Alzheimer's disease therefore varies according to the genes that a person has inherited. For example, a 75-year-old individual with the Apo E2/3 genotype has an 80 per cent chance of not being affected by the disease. However, if that person has inherited Apo E4/4 genotype then they have roughly only a 20 per cent chance of remaining normal.

It is very important to emphasise that knowing someone's Apo E genotypes cannot in any way be taken as a diagnosis of Alzheimer's disease. Some individuals with E4/4 remain normal. There are many other factors that contribute to the final outcome.

Apo E is a susceptibility characteristic. Most people are familiar with susceptibility data in other contexts. For example, it is well known that certain risk factors, such as high cholesterol levels, are associated with an increased risk of heart disease. Being aware of these risks allows the individual to take therapeutic steps to prevent or delay the onset of the disease. Although currently no definitive conclusions can be drawn from Apo E genotyping, medical researchers hope that a cure for DAT will ultimately be available. Nevertheless it needs to be stressed that it is one thing to identify a genetic vulnerability factor and quite another to develop effective and safe new treatments for Alzheimer's disease.

Box 2.3 continued

There is some disagreement over the precise mechanism by which these genetic risk factors are related to the cellular degeneration associated with dementia. One proposed model suggests that the mechanisms through which the brain regenerates malfunctions because of the failure of a protein to make new connections, caused in turn by the apolipoprotein E4 gene products. This results in one of the two characteristic pathological hallmarks of Alzheimer's disease: senile plaques (Cottman 1994). Other researchers have associated cellular degeneration with the development of neurofibrillary tangles (NFTs). Thus the clinical severity of dementia is said to correlate positively with the density of NFTs in parts of the brain. However, the precise mechanism by which NFTs are formed is still not certain.

How common is dementia?

Estimates of the prevalence of dementia vary, but two of the most widely quoted studies suggest the rates shown in Tables 2.2 and 2.3.

We can estimate that roughly 670,000 people in the UK have some form of dementing illness, and of these perhaps 13,000 are aged under 65. Across the country as a whole, there are 500 new cases of dementia per day and 180,000 new cases per year. For an average Health or Local Authority population of 500,000 people in Great Britain, there are likely to be approximately 6000 people suffering from dementia. In addition, there will be a sizeable number of other people who have similar care needs because of the loss of full cognitive functioning, but who do not fit into the strict diagnostic criteria for the dementia syndrome itself.

Table 2.2 Prevalence of dementia (United Kingdom)

	Male	Female	Overall
65–69	3.9%	0.5%	2.1%
70–74	4.1%	2.7%	3.3%
75–79	8.0%	7.9%	8.0%
80 plus	13.2%	20.9%	17.7%

Source: Kay and Bergmann (1980)

Table 2.3 Prevalence of dementia (Europe): age-sex specific rate per 100 population							
Age group							
30–59	60–64	65–69	70–74	75–79	80–84	85–89	90+
Male 0.16	1.58	2.17	4.61	5.04	12.09	18.45	32.00
Female 0.09	0.47	1.10	3.86	6.70	13.50	22.76	32.82

Source: Gordon and Spiker (1997), p.43

Risk factors for DAT and other dementias

Ageing

As Tables 2.2 and 2.3 show, ageing is the largest risk factor for developing a dementing illness, with the prevalence roughly doubling every 5 years between the ages of 65 and 85.

The average age of people has increased steadily over the past 100 years. Better working conditions, improvements in diet and the social and economic changes of the twentieth century mean that, on average, people in Britain can be expected to live 20 or more years longer than would have been the case at the turn of the last century. As a consequence, the total number of people in the UK is set to rise from 56.8 million in 1994 to a peak of 59.4 million around the year 2020. However, as people have also tended to have smaller families over the years, this figure is expected to fall to 57.3 million by 2041.

One of the expected changes that has received most attention is that the proportion of the population who can be thought of as 'old' (say, over the age of 65) and 'very old' (say, over the age of 85) will increase. So over the next 45 years or so (to 2041) the number of people aged over 65 in the UK is likely to increase from 9 million to 14.5 million, while the number of people aged over 85 will more than double, from 1 to 2.2 million. This means that there will be fewer younger people supporting an increasing number of older people in the UK, and that the proportion of the population with an age-related illness will increase.

Family history of Alzheimer's disease

This is a controversial area. Some scientists argue that if there is a family history of dementia in a first degree relative (a sibling or parent) then this increases the risk of developing Alzheimer's disease fourfold, and that in people with two or more affected first degree relatives, the risk increases by seven to eight times. Other studies indicate that there is an increased risk only in the case of pre-senile dementia (dementia which develops before the age of 65).

Family history of Down's syndrome

A family history of Down's syndrome may increase the risk of developing Alzheimer's disease by two to three times.

History of depression

A history of depression more than ten years prior to the onset of AD approximately doubles the risk. The mechanism is unknown, but some studies suggest that the reduced activity of frontal and temporal lobes in depression may make these areas more vulnerable to pathological mechanisms. The relationship between depression and dementia is complex and we will return to this point later in the book.

Oestrogen deficiency

Oestrogen deficiency in post-menopausal women has been implicated in a variety of studies as increasing the risk of Alzheimer's disease and possibly other dementias. This has been demonstrated mostly through studies of women who have had hysterectomies. The reason for this may be oestrogen's influence on nerve growth factor, which supports the neurones that are severely affected in DAT.

Education and occupation

A person with a poor education is about twice as likely to develop dementia due to DAT or vascular disease by the age of 75 as someone who has stayed at school beyond the age of fourteen. This could be due to correlations between health and higher income, better diet and greater access to healthcare. The mechanism by which this occurs may be the strengthening of frequently used brain regions, which may also explain why some people with specific talents or hobbies such as golf, playing music, playing cards or drawing cartoons show preservation of such highly used skills even if they develop DAT. The risk of developing dementia is also reduced for people whose jobs have involved a high level of verbal interaction with other people. However, the fact that Harold Wilson and Ronald Reagan both developed DAT reminds us that, although higher occupational status and levels of education may reduce the risk of developing DAT, it certainly does not eliminate it.

Other possible risks for DAT

Other factors which may increase the risk of DAT include: either severe head injury or repeated blows to the head; a history of high alcohol consumption; a history of heart attacks (especially in women); a family history of Parkinson's disease; and hypothyroidism.

Summary of main points

- Dementia is a term used by psychiatrists to cover a range of symptoms, the most common of which involves the loss of memory. This broad syndrome can then be broken down into particular illnesses, most (but not all) of which are progressive and for which there are no cures. These can be distinguished from the pseudodementias, including depression and delirium which, although producing symptoms that are similar to those of dementia, can be reversed.

- There are three main forms of dementia: Dementia of the Alzheimer's type, multi-infarct dementia and Lewy-body dementia. In addition, there are a number of other illnesses which it is possible to diagnose but which are much less common, including Frontal lobe dementia, Dementia pugilistica and dementia that is associated with various predominantly physical illnesses.

- There are a number of risk factors for dementia. The main risk factor is that of old age; others include a family history of dementia, a personal history of depression and a poor educational and occupational background.

Additional information

Information and support about Alzheimer's disease and other forms of dementia is available from the Alzheimer's Disease Society, Gordon House, 10 Greencoat Place, London SW1P 1PH. Tel: 020 7306 0606; Fax: 020 7306 0808; E-mail: 101762.422 @compuserve.com.

Information and support about Parkinson's disease is available from the Parkinson's Disease Society, 22 Upper Woburn Place, London WC1H 0RA. Tel: 020 7383 3513.

Further information and support about Huntington's disease is available from the Huntington's Disease Association, 108 Battersea High Street, London SW11 3HP. Tel: 020 7223 7000.

CHAPTER 3

The Implications of the Organic Model of Dementia for Dementia Services

I want to say that my mother's true self remains intact, there at the surface of her being, like a feather resting on the surface tension of a glass of water, in the way she listens, nods, rests her hand on her cheek, when we are together. But I stumble along and just stop.

The doctor tries to help me out. 'This seems to matter to you'. 'Because' I say, 'a lot depends on whether people like you treat her as a human being or not'.

She is too clever to rise to this. She deals with beleaguered and hostile relatives all the time. 'This is difficult for you. I know that. My job is to give you the facts'.

'She needs respect,' I say, unsure why I am saying it.

'Of course'. And then she says, reflectively, 'Though who knows what respect means'.

'Just giving her the benefit of the doubt. Just assuming there might be some method in the madness'.

The doctor smiles. 'So act "as if" she is rational. Behave "as if" she knows what she is saying'.

'Exactly'.

I tell her how mother goes in and out of the bathroom five times an hour because she does not want to wet herself but can't tell when she last went to the bathroom. So her strategy is to behave 'as if' she needs to go to the bathroom, whenever the thought occurs to her. There is a method here. This is not just random, panic stricken behaviour. Self-respect is in play here. This is how she manages to avoid making a mess of herself. My voice rises at this point and both of us go silent.

'From a clinical point of view,' she says, taking up the thread, 'disinhibition begins with disintegration in the frontal lobes. Your mother's frontal lobes are not yet affected,' the neurologist goes on, 'which would help to explain why she is continent and why she is gentle'.

'She is gentle,' I say, 'because that's the kind of person that she is'.

'I know how you must feel'.

'Besides,' I say, 'disinhibition is such an ugly word ... Disinhibition suggests that everything is beyond her. Actually she is struggling'.

It is pointless to go on and we both know it. The doctor looks at mother's PET scans and sees a disease of memory function, with a stable name and a clear prognosis. I see an illness of selfhood, without a name or even a clear cause. (Michael Ignatieff 1993, pp.58–60)

In this chapter we will first describe the services available to the person with dementia before moving on, in the second section, to elaborate some concerns about these services.

Let us summarise the organic model or 'standard paradigm' of dementia care as it has come to be known (Kitwood 1990a). Within this paradigm, the 'thing' that is lost in dementia is defined in terms of the person's intellectual, linguistic and cognitive functioning. These losses are said to arise directly from neurological impairment, the origins of which are beginning to be identified as having genetic, molecular and cellular influences. This is, essentially, the representation of dementia in terms of a disease of the brain. The key features of such an approach, in terms of its implications for both the pattern of care provided and the weight given to the internal world of the sufferer, have been summarised in Table 3.1.

As Table 3.1 shows, this understanding of dementia has very important practical implications for the type, range and quality of services that are available to people with dementia.

	Main features	Implications for care management	Implications for the internal world of sufferer
Table 3.1 The standard paradigm of dementia care			
Causation	Only neurological changes are of interest. Cell destruction due to plaques, tangles and vascular destruction. Neurological changes due to biochemical and genetic factors.	The disease is seen as progressive and degenerative, so once established little can be done to affect prognosis. The aim of care is essentially to make life as tolerable as possible.	The internal world is of no consequence to disease process, so it is seen as being of little or no relevance to process of care.
Psychological features	Brain damage, especially alteration in cognitive functioning, personality and memory, are equated with destruction of mind. Dementia is seen as the death of the person.	Emphasis on diagnosis – a need for the assessment of cognitive functioning in order to distinguish between dementias and pseudodementias. The individual is seen as unable to make decisions about their own care.	The internal world of the person with dementia lacks validity, due to the damage to their brain. All necessary decisions should be agreed between professionals and relatives/carers
Symptomology	Many, varied and usually strongly negative. Includes confusion, wandering, disorientation and aggression.	Assessment of problematic behaviours. Medication and behavioural management. Advice and support to carers.	Individual has little meaningful (conscious) control over their actions. The only valid role is that of a 'patient'. Relationships are invalidated.

The assessment of dementia

Medical examination

Dementia, as we have seen, can refer to a broad range of problems. It is therefore important that a complete medical examination be undertaken before a diagnosis is reached (this is often referred to as a 'psychiatric workup'). In a significant proportion of cases these problems are found to be caused not by irreversible damage to the brain but by a reversible cause. Most doctors will want to take a sample of the patient's blood, test the patient's liver and thyroid functioning, find out if there is an infection within the person's urinary tract, look at blood count and so on.

Scans

Occasionally a doctor may ask for a neuroimaging procedure such as a CAT (computed tomography), PET (positron emission tomography), SPECT (single photon emission computed tomography) or MRI (nuclear magnetic resonance imaging) scan. These techniques essentially give a cross-sectional picture of the person's brain, varying in the way they achieve that picture and the type of picture they deliver.

Neuropsychological testing

Where the diagnosis seems to be complex, then often a doctor or psychiatrist will refer the patient to a clinical psychologist for a neuropsychological assessment. Common assessment packages used by clinicians include the CAPE (the Clifton Assessment Procedures for the Elderly) (Pattie and Gilleard 1976) and the Mini-Mental (Folstein, Folstein and McHugh 1975). These are brief screening tests. Lengthier tests sampling a wider range of skills include the MEAMS (the Middlesex Elderly Assessment of Mental State) (Golding 1988); the CAMDEX (the Cambridge Examination for Mental Disorders in the Elderly) (Roth *et al.* 1986; 1988) and the Rivermead Behavioural Memory Test (Wilson, Cockburn and Baddeley 1985; *see also* Twining 1991). These are batteries of tests that assess whether a person has suffered damage to some or all of their intellectual functioning. As dementia is taken to be an illness that affects almost every aspect of a person's intellectual and emotional functioning rather than specific or focal areas of the brain (i.e. a global problem), so these assessment tests are very general, and look to see whether a range of abilities have been affected.

Despite these techniques, the assessment of dementia still relies on the subjective interpretation of the data, albeit by experienced clinicians. Mistakes do occur, and all clinicians would say that definitive diagnosis is only possible at post-mortem, when the brain cells can be examined. Furthermore, the diagnosis of the different specific forms of dementia is still very difficult even for experienced clinicians.

Caring for a dementia sufferer

As the dementia progresses to a severe level the person becomes unable to live without help. Loss of memory, the most prominent feature, leads to an inability to carry out 'higher' functions such as preparing meals, paying bills or shopping. Some patients gradually become unable to cope unaided with basic functions such as toileting, washing and eating. Some sufferers will wander out of their homes while others may leave the gas or taps on. Many, due to their advanced age, have co-existing physical illnesses which complicate their care.

Yet despite these problems, the vast majority of dementia sufferers are cared for at home by their husband, wife, son or daughter. This places an enormous stress on their 'carers', most of whom are relatively old themselves, often have their own physical health problems, and tend to become cut-off from their normal sources of support. Most carers are women who are looking after their husbands, brothers, fathers or fathers-in-law.

The progressive cognitive impairment found in an older person with dementia presents unique problems to those who are involved in caring for them. For instance, carers may find the loss of human understanding from those they have known for many years very difficult to cope with. Aggressive behaviour, wandering and dangerous forgetfulness may develop. These problems are all the more painful to see when they occur not in a stranger but in one's husband, wife, father or mother. The person with advanced or severe dementia may need almost constant supervision to ensure their safety.

Many carers rate their greatest problems as:

- not being able to leave their relative on his/her own for even one hour
- the relative's lack of concern for personal hygiene
- the relative's inability to take part in a conversation with the family
- sitting around doing nothing
- the relative wandering around the house at night.

Consequently, it is important that the statutory health and social services and the many different voluntary groups that are involved give support to carers before a crisis becomes an emergency. Although service provision varies widely across the UK, various forms of day and respite care and other forms of support for carers are likely to be available.

The early identification of dementia

In recent years there has been an increase in the amount of service and policy attention to the early identification of dementia and to the provision of appropriate support at this time (see Jackson and Wonson 1987; David 1991; Burningham 1992; Duff and Peach 1994; Gatz 1995; LaBarge and Trtanj 1995; Gibson and Moniz-Cook 1996). The Alzheimer's Disease Society (ADS), in their 1995 annual campaign and report (Alzheimer's Disease

Society 1995), reinforced this need for services, and the diagnoses, to be 'right from the start'. In short, the ADS contend that an early approach to case identification gives people with dementia and their families time to adjust to the diagnosis and plan for their respective futures – a practice position also suggested explicitly in the recent Social Services Inspectorate (SSI) and Department of Health (DoH) joint report (Social Services Inspectorate/Department of Health 1996).

In theory at least, an early diagnosis can act as a trigger for an assessment of need for the person with dementia under the Community Care legislation (Department of Health 1990) and, independently for the carer(s), under the Carers (Recognition and Services) Act (Department of Health 1995) and its accompanying practice guidelines (Department of Health 1996). Whilst it is difficult to argue against the underlying ethos of this approach, Keady (1996), in a review of the literature on the experience of dementia, suggested that confirming an early diagnosis of dementia is an extremely complex act which involves the exclusion of other symptomatology, including benign senile forgetfulness, age-associated memory impairment, depressive pseudodementia and other underlying physical causes such as normal pressure hydrocephalus, cerebral tumour or drug toxicity. Moreover, few studies, if any, are concerned with or about the impact of cognitive assessment on the individuals themselves and the context in which the assessment takes place.

Early diagnosis: policy considerations

To date most research attention and service provision has been targeted at people in the more advanced stages of dementia, at which point services can be visible and focused on supporting the carer (for carer-centred literature reviews *see* Morris, Morris and Britton 1988; Kuhlman *et al.* 1991; Vitaliano, Young and Russo 1991; Knight, Lutzky and Macofsky-Urban 1993).

The 1980s and early 1990s saw the development of memory clinics in most major cities. These aimed to provide an earlier diagnosis (Wright and Lindesay 1995; Gilliard and Gwilliam 1996), and to provide memory support to people with dementia (Zarit, Gallagher and Kramer 1981; Karlsson *et al.* 1989; Woods 1994; for a review *see* Wilson 1994). Unfortunately, many memory clinics seemed little more than entrance points for drug trials, and did not offer long-term help and intervention.

Thus, while memory clinics may at a *prima facie* level appear to be a panacea for the late identification of memory impairment, their effectiveness in meeting the reported needs of their user groups remains open to question (Wright and Lindesay 1995; Gilliard and Gwilliam 1996), particularly in the amount of advice they give on how to actually live with the memory problem(s) (*see* Hill *et al.* 1995 and Bender 1996c for reviews of the ethical and theoretical issues).

With regard to the sufferer, Rice and Warner (1994) suggested that people with a diagnosed mild cognitive impairment/dementia had a right to be informed of their diagnosis, despite the concerns that this may pose to their family supporter(s) (Maguire *et al.* 1996). A literature review of the merits of early diagnosis concluded that 'there is unanimous agreement in the literature that an early, accurate diagnosis would benefit' (Downs *et al.* 1994), but then found little empirical support for the claim (Goldsmith 1996). In a similar vein, O'Connor *et al.* (1991), in a study of services and service improvement in Cambridge, found that early professional intervention increased the rate of admission to residential care, with 64 per cent of those living alone receiving extra support, compared to 8 per cent of the controls, within two years, p=0.004. (For a more positive outcome, using Intensive Case Management, *see* Challis *et al.* 1997.)

The move to early diagnosis was recently highlighted again in an informative report which reviewed the practice of assessment for older people with dementia living in the community (Social Services Inspectorate/ Department of Health 1996). This report was based on one-day visits to five local authorities in the summer of 1995.

From the areas visited in the report, satisfactory solutions were not forthcoming, and older people with dementia were only identified in the community once their problems became severe, thus limiting the range of services, intervention and support that could be provided. As usual, it was social or familial disturbance that triggered action, not its cause – cognitive loss. If cognitive loss is undisturbing it will often, if not usually, fail to reach the public service domain. Furthermore, the annual 75+ health checks were seen in the report as a 'good tool' for identifying dementia at an early stage, although few authorities had progressed this idea into a formal assessment procedure.

In common with most other reports of this type (e.g. Alzheimer's Disease Society 1995) the authors placed the emphasis upon the philosophical need for early case identification, and paid little attention to the underlying processes involved, i.e. the context and environment, and the reliability of brief screening tools used in the assessment procedure. Interestingly, the authors could find few articles on the subjective experience of cognitive assessment, and those references which could be traced give rise for considerable concern (Dahlberg and Jaffe 1977; Davis 1989; McGowin 1993). For instance, in their separate written accounts of 'journies' into Alzheimer's disease, both Davis (1989) and McGowin (1993) rarely mention professional interventions and when they do, it is in terms of frustration and hostility. In particular, both authors expressed their distress at:

- the time it took to establish a diagnosis
- being kept in the dark over the outcome of assessment investigations
- the lack of dedicated support
- the inadequate supply of information.

In the United Kingdom, Keady and Nolan (1995a) suggest that people with dementia at this early stage require distinct and separate services. In agreement with Froggatt (1988) they propose a role for an 'independent confidante' who can act as a buffer between the experience of dementia and the desire of the individual to somehow protect their supporter from its ongoing impact. However, for this situation to materialise, there is an urgent need to consider both the environment and biographical context in which assessment takes place, and the expectations of the process by the people with cognitive impairment themselves. We will return to this issue in a later chapter, in which we outline a more consumer-friendly version of the assessment procedure.

The development of memory enhancing drugs

By mid1998 two drugs were being marketed in the United Kingdom which, it is claimed, improve the cognitive functioning of people with DAT. These are Aricept which has recently been approved in both the US and the UK for use on patients with mild to moderately severe DAT, and Exelon.

Aricept (Donepezil hydrochloride)

Aricept seems to be effective in enhancing or maintaining the cognitive functioning of about 40 per cent of the DAT sufferers to whom it is given. Aricept may improve the DAT patient's ability to perform a variety of everyday living skills. The usual dose is a single 5 mg tablet given once a day. A 10 mg tablet is available, and although more side effects may be seen with the higher dose, this can be attempted after a four-to-six-week period. Side effects, when they do occur, are usually thought to be transient and are primarily related to the gastrointestinal tract, with nausea, diarrhoea and vomiting being the most commonly reported.

Aricept works by having an effect on one of the chemical pathways in the brain that is involved in laying down memories (as well as other cognitive abilities) and which is damaged in the early stages of DAT. These pathways are found in the cerebral cortex and the basal ganglia, and use acetylcholine to enable messages to pass from one nerve cell to the next. After it has been released into the synapse or the gap between the two cells, the acetylcholine is destroyed by a substance called acetylcholinesterase. Aricept works by stopping the acetylcholinesterase from destroying the neurochemical transmitter, thereby helping to build up supplies of the transmitter between the nerves. For people with DAT whose pathways have been affected, this can be an effective way of helping them to pass messages between cells and thereby retain as much cognitive functioning as possible for as long as possible. Exelon's formulation and method of working in the brain is essentially similar to that of Aricept.

Unfortunately, DAT involves much more than just damage to one set of pathways, and as the disease progresses so the ability of these drugs to reduce the effects of the damage to these pathways is reduced.

Aricept and Exelon are just the first of many drugs that will appear over the next few years. Other drugs are being developed, such as ampakines which enhance the action of glutamate, a different neurochemical pathway to cholinesterase, but one that is also involved in cognitive functioning.

Problems with the use of memory enhancing drugs

There are, unfortunately, downsides to these drugs which have made many doctors and clinicians rather cautious about their use. As we have described, Aricept does not help everybody, even in cases where the dementia sufferer has been carefully assessed as potentially suitable. There is a danger, then, that many people will have their hopes raised only to find that the drug is not of help to them or to their loved ones. There are cost implications – Aricept costs around £900 to £1000 per person, per year, at 1998 prices. Given the number of people who might be suitable for a trial of the drug, then in the UK, overall, the NHS may need to find another £25 million per year to pay for this treatment. Consequently, many health authorities may not be able to afford to prescribe it without an increase in their drug budgets. Moreover, using the drug requires patients to be assessed before and during their treatment to see if they are suitable and whether, if they are prescribed the drug, they improve. Such assessments are time-consuming and expensive, and will again require additional resources.

A more fundamental limitation of these drugs is that they do not directly affect the disease process itself, but act to enhance the person's remaining ability to learn and remember. They do not, therefore, represent a cure – at best they are a way of extending the course of the illness, of delaying but not preventing decline. As these drugs do not directly affect the DAT disease process, but instead act to enhance a person's ability to remember, it may be that relatively soon there will be pressure to license these, or other similar drugs, for use with people who do not have a dementing illness – with older people with very mild, normal forms of forgetfulness, for example, and perhaps with students preparing to sit exams. Many psychologists and others are concerned that the development of Aricept and other memory drugs may be the start of a process of medicalising and pathologising normal everyday life. Many would argue that we are in danger of seeing a similar phenomenon to that which accompanied the marketing of Prozac, in which many were seduced by promises of a miracle cure that took away unhappiness without any side effects.

Aspirin

The medical treatment of vascular dementia involves trying to treat the underlying medical risks for vascular disease and stroke. One way of doing this is through the use of anti-coagulents such as Aspirin and Ticlopidine. These do not improve memory performance, but can help to prevent the build-up of blood clots that subsequently lead to strokes. Where the person is able to exercise, the cardiovascular equivalent of walking 5 miles per week improves cardiac output and efficiency.

The changing face of service provision: a 'rising tide' of dementia?

Let us try to summarise the practical implications of the organic model. Table 3.2 lists the main effects.

Table 3.2 The service implications of the organic model
1. The person with Alzheimer's is treated as a non-person.
2. The disease must be understood as irreversible.
3. It suggests strongly that loss of control is a major feature of dementia.
4. It encourages, rather than provides scientific evidence for, therapeutic nihilism.
5. It discourages any interest in the subjective experience of the sufferer.
6. There is too much emphasis on assessment, especially of memory.
7. It simplifies the carer role.
8. It sees the only hope as lying in drug advances.
9. It has worrying social implications.

In Chapter 2 we outlined how the average age of the population of the UK, like that of most Western industrialised countries, is projected to increase. The realisation that these demographic changes will have significant effects has prompted both major political parties in the UK to implement a series of important reforms to the overall organisation of the welfare state, including a major overhaul of the pension system.

At least until the year 2020, the additional cost of caring for older people is unlikely to significantly exceed the growth of GNP. However, the proportion of overall expenditure devoted to older people (including those older people with mental illnesses) will need to increase. In addition, older people from ethnic minority groups may become especially disadvantaged. For instance, within the Pakistani and Bangladeshi communities, there are currently relatively high numbers of people in the 50–59 age group. Moreover, as we have seen, dementia is closely associated with ageing; therefore as the number of old people in the UK increases, so we can expect the number of people with dementia to increase significantly.

In this chapter we have outlined some of the issues that have driven service delivery to dementia sufferers and their carers over the last decade or more. Our argument has been that these services are based around the medical model of dementia, the standard paradigm, which views dementia as simply the destruction of the brain and thus ignores both the subjective experiences of the dementia sufferer and their place within a social world. We would suggest that the model has dangerous implications for people diagnosed as having dementia. A society which today treats certain kinds of people as if they do not exist psychologically may tomorrow treat them as if they do not deserve to exist physically.

As long as the organic paradigm remains unchallenged, the therapeutic nihilism explicit in the paradigm (that nothing can be achieved till the wonder drug cometh) will make it likely that people with dementia will be stripped of their personhood when they receive the diagnosis. At its worst, this leads to people with dementia being placed within institutions, almost as goods are placed in a warehouse, with a quality of care that is barely acceptable (Miller and Gwynne 1972). As a result of Care in the Community there are fewer long-stay beds, and people are going into hospital later and for shorter periods. In the case of dementia, this means that more people are entering 'long-stay' wards or nursing homes with severe loss of ability and behavioural disorders than formerly. Of course, many dementia sufferers are going into nursing homes. While there are some exceptions, it is hard to imagine that these often provide a stimulating or individualistic environment, given the low levels of external supervision. Moreover, the high use of untrained staff found in the field of dementia care is hardly surprising if any more sophisticated efforts requiring trained staff are regarded as a waste of time.

Because of its denial of or lack of interest in emotional suffering, the current organic paradigm has to be supplemented with a more humane approach. We cannot continue to walk away from the suffering being inflicted by neglect on people with dementia. We cannot leave their 'care' to neurology and neuropsychology, because the evidence of the quality of the care resulting from their approach is all too clear. There have to be theoretical alternatives that more closely mirror the reality of the individual and thus offer more relevant and effective care; in Part Two, we start to elaborate these alternatives.

In the next chapter we will move on to provide a critique of this organic model of dementia and its implications for service delivery. The need to base our services around the subjective experiences of dementia sufferers becomes increasingly important in the context of the demographic changes that are occurring and also the introduction of new drugs that will delay, without preventing, the cognitive decline of dementia.

CHAPTER 4

The Limitations of the Organic Model

The organic model of dementia

As we described in the previous chapters, dementia research has been dominated by the psychiatric or medical approach to dementia – what Tom Kitwood has called the 'standard paradigm' of dementia care. There are major gaps in the evidence for the validity of this approach. In this chapter we outline some of its main shortcomings.

Let us start by considering what the approach has achieved. There have been important recent developments, for example drugs such as Aricept, the finding of genetic risk factors for developing particular forms of dementia and the identification of the cellular precipitants of the disease.

Yet it has not only been in medical research that significant developments have occurred. At the same time, increasing numbers of psychological and psychotherapeutic approaches to dementia have emerged, and these psychosocial developments have been collectively termed 'the new culture of dementia care' (Kitwood and Benson 1995). At first sight it might seem odd that at the very moment that the organic paradigm begins to fulfil its promise by bringing forth drugs with such potential to postpone cognitive decline, this way of thinking about dementia should be attacked most strongly. However, the development of memory enhancing drugs, on its own, does not prove that the standard paradigm is the only way of thinking about people with dementia. Anyway, at present these drugs simply alleviate some of the symptoms of dementia and do not represent a cure.

Criticisms of the organic model

Over the last ten years significant changes in how we think about dementia have occurred. Our understanding of dementia has moved away from a narrow focusing on brain functioning and cognitive loss, and the dementia sufferer is now seen both as existing within a social world and as having a lifetime of experiences and knowledge. In this chapter we will present a brief overview of the range of criticisms that have been made of the organic model. These are listed in Box 4.1.

Box 4.1 Criticisms of the organic model

1. The impact of the social world is ignored

2. The experiences of people with dementia are neglected

3. The diagnosis of dementia can be unreliable

4. The link between clinical and neurological change is unclear

5. Dementia can be better understood as a disability than as a disease

6. Alternative concepts of memory and memory loss are ignored, see p.86

7. The stage model of dementia is inadequate

8. Old age has been medicalised

9. People experience dementia within a lifetime of experiences

10. People with dementia are seen as a burden.

The impact of the social world is ignored

Although many researchers and clinicians have expressed concerns about aspects of the medical approach to dementia, arguably the most significant critique from the UK was published in the early 1990s by Tom Kitwood, a social psychologist at the University of Bradford. Since then Kitwood has gone on to develop an important model of dementia care – one to which we will continue to refer throughout this book.

Tom Kitwood's criticism of the standard paradigm is essentially that dementia sufferers are social beings. What he and we mean by this is that all of us live and are cared for within a social world of relationships and communication. It is through these relationships that we establish a sense of who we are – our identity, or as Tom Kitwood has referred to it, our personhood. People with dementia will be best able to hold on to a positive sense of their own identity if the people around them treat them with respect and consideration.

Kitwood and Bredin (1992) have argued powerfully that once someone has been diagnosed as having a progressive memory loss they are subjected to a debilitating onslaught both from within and from the outside world. For instance, they can be *disempowered* (things are done for them that they are able to do for themselves); *intimidated* (e.g. through the use of scans, psychological tests and seemingly irrelevant questions); and *invalidated* (the subjectivity of the dementia sufferer is ignored or overlooked). Thus the malignant social psychology surrounding the individual attacks his or her personhood through a dialectical process whereby a gradual neurological impairment interacts with a process of disempowerment, a loss of self-esteem and the stereotyping assumptions of others.

Dementia often causes a person's sense of identity to be under threat, so it is no surprise that much of 'the new culture of dementia care' has been devoted to considerations of how the delivery of care to people with dementia can be organised so that their sense of self can be preserved for as long as possible.

The experiences of people with dementia are neglected

The medical model or psychiatric view sees dementia predominantly in terms of the loss of brain tissue and, stemming from this, the loss of cognitive functioning, emotional control and personality. Those clinical changes that occur are viewed as the consequences of damage to specific parts of the brain. It is frequently said that emotional control and personality depend upon the areas at the front of the brain, while language is controlled by areas generally found on the left hand side. Damage to either of these areas of the brain leads to problems in controlling behaviour or expressing oneself. However, the reverse is not necessarily true: it is not the case that if a person has problems expressing or controlling him- or herself that these problems were inevitably caused by damage to their brain (and it is through their behaviour that we know people).

As we have seen in Chapter 3, the standard paradigm representation of what is lost as a result of the dementing process carries with it significant implications for the types of services and interventions that are considered appropriate. For instance, as dementia is represented in terms of the loss of cognitive functioning, one of the most frequently reported psychological interventions has been Reality Orientation, which it is hoped will increase such functioning (Holden and Woods 1995). The psychologist, or more generally a relatively untrained nursing assistant or carer, acts as an external prompt to the dementia sufferer's waning intellectual powers. The dementia sufferer is thus seen as a dysfunctional learner, with the most appropriate therapy thought to be one which compensates for these losses.

However, these ideas about dementia can only be part of the picture. For instance, when we work with a dementia sufferer, we are not just dealing with someone whose brain functioning has been undermined by the disease process, but with a person who has had a lifetime of experiences and learning. As well as thinking of dementia sufferers as people whose brains have been damaged, we can also see them as having an active mental life and as social beings – as people struggling to come to terms with the changes taking place inside and around them.

Yet all too often dementia care services view the person with dementia as having nothing meaningful to say about their condition; it is as if they have no valid feelings, no personhood and no sense of agency. Conditions, once above humane, can be changed without reference to the people concerned, who can be treated, assessed and medicated without thought of obtaining meaningful consent. The only valid role left for the individual is that of a patient, and all relationships are transformed into those appropriate for this new status. Opportunities to continue to be a mother, lover, husband or brother are lost, partly because of the effects of the illness itself and partly because of the way in which social relationships are transformed.

The assumption that people with dementia are almost non-people means that it is hard to arouse practitioner interest in exploring their subjective world. What are they feeling? How do their feelings change over time? What is it like to be assessed, to be in a day unit for people with dementia or to be on an Elderly Mentally Impaired (EMI) ward? We have very little under-standing of what it is like to have dementia largely because this has not seemed to be an important question to answer. In the standard paradigm, the internal world of dementia sufferers is almost irrelevant.

Compare this with going to hospital to see a cancer specialist. Imagine that the doctor gets all the results, calls you and your partner in and addresses all his or her remarks to your partner while you sit there. You would find this quite unacceptable and if you complained your complaint would be upheld.

The diagnosis of dementia can be unreliable

As we have described in the last two chapters, the psychiatric system of classifying illnesses rests on a central proposition: that it is possible to distinguish normal from abnormal processes. In attempting to diagnose dementia, clinicians therefore assume that there is a hard and fast distinction between normal and abnormal ageing. However, there appears to be no clear boundary for the diagnosis of dementia. This is because the cognitive decline found in those people who are given a diagnosis of dementia lies on the same continuum as that occurring in the general ageing population. It is particularly difficult to diagnose early or mild dementia, since other psychological conditions such as anxiety and depression can produce cognitive profiles which are similar to those associated with the milder stages of this disease. (Those illnesses that can produce similar cognitive errors are called pseudodementias.)

The response to these diagnostic difficulties is usually to refer to all diagnoses of dementia made on the basis of test performances and clinical presentations as provisional. Typically, it is claimed that definite diagnoses are possible, but only when a sample of brain tissue can be examined under the microscope – and of course, this is generally only possible once the person has died. Thus it is often assumed that although the clinical assessment of dementia may be subjective and difficult to define, the changes that occur within the brain in Alzheimer's disease are widely agreed upon. In actual fact, this is not really the case:

> A number of important points emerge with respect to the differential diagnosis and classification of dementia-producing conditions. Although diseases such as Alzheimer's and Pick's are defined in terms of neuropathology, and it is the goal of all serious researchers to have their clinical diagnoses validated by autopsy (or biopsy) examination, there is surprisingly little consensus among pathologists in terms of what are the critical features and the quantity and/or distribution of these necessary to justify diagnosis of a particular condition. Thus the supposedly gold standard for diagnosis is no more objectively defined than the clinical criteria. The neuropathological criteria need to be standardised, with agreement on minimal counts of particular morphological features required in specified areas of the brain. Such standards have been proposed for AD (Khachaturian, 1985) but are not in general use. The lack of well defined and widely accepted criteria is clearly an impediment to research in this area. (Hart and Semple 1994, p.43)

The link between clinical and neurological change is unclear

There is, then, surprisingly little consensus amongst scientists on the critical neurological features and the quantity and/or distribution of these necessary to justify diagnosis of a particular condition. There are almost as many problems in reaching a diagnosis from direct post-mortem examination of the brain as there are in achieving a diagnosis from clinical evidence. Part of the problem results from symptom heterogeneity – that the symptoms described in the textbooks are apparently sharp and clear, whereas, typically, those encountered in the clinical setting are blurred, and far more varied.

There are also other problems with establishing a link between the behaviour and symptoms of dementia sufferers and an underlying neurological disease process. First, there is no clear-cut link between the plaques and neurofibrillary tangles (NFTs) that are associated with DAT and the clinical symptoms of dementia. For instance, NFTs can be seen in almost all older (and some younger) people. Thus one study has identified that 75 per cent of individuals aged between 55 and 64 are affected by NFTs (Ulrich 1985). Indeed, post-mortem examinations indicate that individuals can have symptoms of dementia without great neurological damage. It is thus possible to have neurological damage without apparent symptoms and symptoms without damage. Therefore, it is clear that 'the pathological changes occurring in dementia of Alzheimer type are not unique to this condition, but found also in the normal ageing brain' (Hart and Semple 1994, p.44).

Second, even if we do find a statistical correlation between the clinical symptoms of dementia and neurological damage, we still will not completely understand the nature of that association. It may be that both symptoms and damage are caused by either a third agent or an interaction between individual, psychosocial and many other factors. Thus data on risk factors indicates that there is some form of genetic involvement at a predisposing level, with other risk factors such as education, occupation and social class also being involved in the genesis of Alzheimer's disease. Hence the existence of NFTs or other pathological features does not rule out the involvement of psychological and social factors in the development and maintenance of dementia.

Finally, we must also remember that the brain is incredibly plastic. Professor John Lober published a paper in the respectable journal *Developmental Medicine and Child Neurology* in the mid 1960s. It showed a CAT scan of a man with a very small brain size. This man had obtained 'a first class honours degree in economics, mathematics and computer studies and possesses an IQ of 126' (Paterson 1980).

The importance of such work is that it shows that functions normally associated with one part of the brain or one site can be transferred, albeit to a limited extent, to other sites, and this is quite often seen in brain injury cases such as road traffic accidents. If we accept this – and we don't have much choice – then it may be theoretically possible that a similar transfer of functions, to at least some degree, might be achievable with Alzheimer's disease and other dementias.

The plasticity of the brain may, to some extent, account for clinical cases in which someone who appears to have the pattern of symptoms consistent with dementia does not deteriorate in the way that might be expected from such a diagnosis. Standard medical definitions of dementia, in which the disease is understood to be irreversible, find such examples difficult to deal with. This is because if all the changes in people with dementia that we see are caused by brain cell death, then the progress of this disease will be seen as irreversible. There is, however, evidence to the contrary. Not only are there the relatively frequent examples of cases which are subsequently redefined as misdiagnoses, but without in any way carrying out an exhaustive search we found evidence of positive change in McPherson and Tregaskis (1985) in Dundee, Ames *et al.* (1988) among residents of old people's homes in Camden, and Bayles, Tomoeda and Trosset (1993) in Arizona. Similarly, attempts have been made to reverse or at least slow down the assumed inevitable deterioration. Examples, again by no means exhaustive, include Brody *et al.* (1971) and Annerstedt (1994), who compared people with dementia living in group living (GL) situations with those living in traditional institutions (TI). On the basis of the favourable outcome for those in group living, Annerstedt summarised: 'Offering GL care as an alternative to TI might raise the quality of life in the demented elderly for a period of 2–2.5 years' (p.372). More controversially, Louis Blank gives clear evidence in *Alzheimer's Challenged and Conquered?* (1995) that he was so diagnosed, and then says he cured himself. Similarly, Tom Kitwood, in one study, asked like-minded workers for examples of what he has described as 'rementia' and established 45 reports of such positive changes (Kitwood 1996).

We still have the same problem that Alzheimer and Kraepelin struggled with and which we described in Chapter 1: that of separating the mass of clinical cases into specific disease categories. Arguably, we should be looking at functional loss rather than at specific disease categories. If we focus on functional losses, the problem of the unreliability of disease categories disappears – we don't need them. So instead of seeking to distinguish depression from dementia we should treat the functional symptoms of memory loss and emotional sadness.

Dementia can be better understood as a disability than as a disease

One of the main professional tasks for people working with dementia sufferers and their families is that of assessment to find out the extent and perhaps the type of damage, and the speed at which this damage is advancing. Many nursing, occupational therapy and clinical psychology interventions aim to answer these and only these questions.

Much of the focus of the assessment of people with dementia is devoted to answering the psychiatric or medical question: 'What illness, if any, does this person suffer from?' In practical terms, however, the most important questions to answer concern what skills are affected and what the person needs in order to be able to function at their highest levels. When we work with someone with dementia we need to know how to communicate with them and how to organise their care so that they feel comforted and enabled to be the best that they can be. These questions require answers that the standard psychiatric assessment simply cannot provide.

Rather than assessing patients with the aim of establishing the form and level of their cognitive impairments, we suggest that assessment of disability should be the first objective, and the mental or physical causes should be uncovered next. A suitable informant such as their carer may be the best judge of the nature of the disability. This procedure is especially important when it comes to planning services, as it would show which and what level of services people with dementia actually require, clarify the implications of dementia for estimates of active-life-expectancy and increase comparability between different research studies (Kay 1994). This approach would also avoid confusing the issue by deducing an underlying physical cause.

Marshall (1996) outlines a number of advantages of seeing dementia as a disability rather than as an illness, in particular for the design of buildings. This approach is characterised by an emphasis on the disabled sufferer having an impaired memory, impaired reasoning, impaired ability to learn, a high level of stress and an acute sensitivity to the social and built environment. All of this leads the person with dementia to have difficulty in adapting to new situations. The appropriate design of buildings can compensate for this disability to some degree.

Alternative concepts of memory and memory loss are ignored

Memory loss has long been viewed as one, if not the major, symptom of dementia (Miller and Morris 1993). The ability to remember is typically seen in terms of a storage model of memory: a fixed capacity container into which memories can be placed and from which they can be retrieved. This model dates from at least the time of Aristotle, who described memory through the analogy of a wax plate onto which a mark could be placed; the force with which the mark was made and the firmness of the wax determined how long the impression lasted.

The storage model of memory is established within both professional and lay usage. Thus the principal concern of many mental health workers has been to make an assessment of how well this storage and retrieval process is functioning, with the recalled memories being assessed in terms of their truthfulness or veracity. The issue of verifiability that has thus come to dominate the area has two strands. If individuals can be shown to have a reduced ability to remember what they have just been told, and if their memories can thus be shown to be unreliable, then they can be taken, as people, to lack the competence to place meaning on life.

The employment of a model in which there is assumed to be a number of distinctively different types of 'memory' that are capable of being measured objectively has constrained the study of remembering. Psychologists and others have become the 'experts' on memory, with the accounts of the individuals concerned taken to be of interest only inasmuch as they provide evidence that relates to this underlying deficit. From this basis, whatever people have to say about the past tends to be interpreted in terms of the storage model of memory: changes in narratives or the repeated use of similar narratives are represented as confabulation or perseveration. Both are taken as further evidence of neurological impairment, and the significance of this talk is thus narrowly defined, with alternative possibilities discounted.

Recently, social psychologists have suggested an alternative framework within which to think about memory: a discursive action model (e.g. Edwards, Potter and Middleton 1992). This model emphasises the context within which the remembering occurs and the function to which talk about the past is put. Thus the social process in which memories are created and gain meaning becomes of enormous importance.

Middleton and Edwards (1990) propose that memory has the function of providing a narrative that helps the person make sense of their life and communicate with others. They are therefore much less concerned with the veracity of an account, and would be even if it were possible to compare the recollected account of an event with an exact version of how things were at that time. Instead, the discursive action model involves the study of remembering as people actually do it, as reflected in their talk about the past (Middleton and Edwards 1990). It is through talk about the past that people are able to establish a version of themselves as social beings, move others towards accepting their version of events, or create a shared sense of belonging. Discursive approaches orientate us towards examining the function rather than the form of 'memory'.

The standard psychological way of conceptualising the process of remembering in terms of the reliability of a person's memory has prevented us from asking some important questions. Instead of being concerned with 'truthfulness' we could ask questions such as 'What is the function of this talk?', 'Within which social contexts does talk stay the same or change?' and 'What are the effects of others responding to this talk as if it were meaningless?'

Cheston (1996) has described how individuals with dementia are able to both talk about the past as a way of making sense of their present experiences and comment upon this process. For example, one person may use his experience of being at Dunkirk as evidence that he can cope now; another may claim/request treatment as a person of substance because of their previous employment. Two of the people with dementia that he reports describe recreating the past through talk as an active coping strategy to overcome feelings of being useless and make sense of the world. Similarly, Buchanan and Middleton (1994) have examined how within a reminiscence group, talk about the past, and in particular talk about occasions on which participants have been able to help other people, fulfils a number of functions. Participants use such talk, for instance, to establish a shared sense of social identity and as a means of establishing their entitlement to care.

The stage model of dementia is inadequate

Although the term 'dementia' is frequently used to refer to a collection of distinct illnesses, these illnesses are said nevertheless to share some common features, one of which is that the sufferer progresses through a series of stages. For example, Reisberg et al. (1982) describe six stages and then further buttress this definition of reality by creating the Global Deterioration Scale to define which stage a person is in. Similarly, multi-infarct dementia is commonly described as developing in a step-like manner, with mini-strokes (infarcts) and plateau stages during which the competence level holds until the next infarct.

But are these regularities easily observable or are they in the minds of clinicians, who, espousing the organic model, want (and need) evidence of a developing disease? One study by Gubrium (1987) found that although health care professionals working with people with dementia spoke to carers and relatives about the illness of dementia as progressing in a series of stages, they were much more vague when asked about specific individuals. When they had to talk about a particular person, then instead of identifying that person as being at a particular stage they frequently said that it was impossible to tell or that the person had good days and bad days, and so on. Stages, then, seemed to apply only to the general concept of dementia and not to particular people. Gubrium suggested that because these descriptions of stages implied detailed observation and measurement, they served to link the study of dementia to high-prestige methods and areas of science – they were a way in which the physician could claim to have access to a higher level of knowledge and expertise.

There are remarkably few longitudinal studies of dementia – studies in which people with dementia are studied over a long period of time. This is important because it is not clear that everyone with early dementia will necessarily get worse; and it is certainly not true that they will get worse/decline at the same rate.

Let us be reasonable and agree that most people with dementia will get worse over time *but at very different rates*. As a psychiatrist colleague, Arik Solytjiak, observed, 'they'll get worse but we don't know and can't tell how far and how fast' (personal communication). If this is the case – and it is hard to argue against it – then what is left of the stages model? Some people go from being mildly impaired to severely impaired in a matter of months. Do they go through visible and recordable stages? Or is all that we can say that their degree of difficulty increases dramatically?

So, could it be that the concept of stages results from an averaging out of many people whose dementia status has changed? This averaging out produces a reasonably smooth line which is in turn been chopped up into stages. Figures 3.1 and 3.2 demonstrate how this artefact is produced.

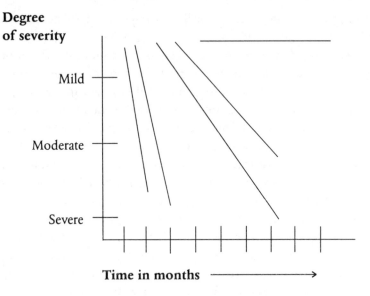

Each line represents one patient's change over time

Figure 3.1 Movement of five individuals with dementia from diagnosis as having mild dementia
Source: Bender and Wainwright (1998a)

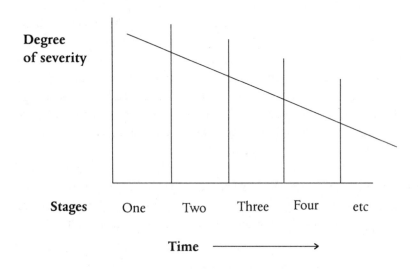

Figure 3.2 Smoothed-out averaging of the five patients' change in Figure 3.1
Source: Bender and Wainwright (1998a)

It is because people do not go through all the assumed stages of dementia that from time to time a person will arrive at hospital with very severe cognitive deficits but no history of any involvement with health professionals. The clinician will ask when the relative first noted something different. The relative, who is also using a (stages of) disease model, will say 'Two years ago', and this probably irrelevant piece of behaviour is taken as the start of the disease process.

It is more sensible to say the person never passed through any stages. He or she experienced a severe change from normal cognitive functioning to cognitive damage. He or she did not go through any stages – quickly or otherwise – because there were not any stages to go through.

Old age has been medicalised

Medical and psychiatric diagnostic systems necessarily focus upon areas of functioning in which people can be defined as being deficient. This generates a language in which individuals are reduced to the status of patients or people with areas of incompetence. This is true of dementia: to talk about someone as having a dementing illness is necessarily to focus on areas of their performance in which they are found wanting, and to ascribe that performance deficit to a state of illness.

It has not always been this way. Not so long ago the problems that we now refer to as being produced by an illness such as DAT were viewed as a consequence of ageing – as being typical of senility. Thus the American sociologist Jaber Gubrium (1986; 1987) has argued that images of ageing as a general period of decay have been transformed into images of a disease – of an illness that some will suffer but not others. The implication is that this disease can be avoided – that it will affect some people and not others and that it is potentially curable. Gubrium argues that this is just one of the changes that society has made to remove ageing from the realm of nature and place it within the realm of science.

People experience dementia within a lifetime of experiences

Just as each of us is a unique individual, so every person will respond to dementia in their own unique way. Some people will experience it as a challenge to be overcome, while others will be overcome with terror and fear. We might expect that those individuals who can be thought of as being, in some way, more psychologically healthy before the onset of the illness will be able to deal with the process of neurological damage in more adaptive ways than can those who are psychologically weaker. The picture that we will see of someone with dementia, then, is the result not only of neurological deterioration, but of the person's psychological health and well-being.

Miesen and Jones (1997) relate the resurfacing of psychic pain in dementia to traumas experienced earlier in life, for instance during war. They argue that the experience of alienation from others and ultimately from oneself that dementia brings is essentially similar to earlier traumas. Those who have been unable to deal successfully with earlier traumatic experiences are likely to have even greater difficulty adjusting to dementia. We will return to these issues, and in particular the role played by a person's first experiences of being parented or looked after (often referred to as attachment relationships), in a later chapter.

People with dementia are seen as a burden

Dementia is a disease like no other disease. From being competent, thinking people, dementia sufferers are gradually reduced to a state that may appear to be one of almost complete disintegration. The emotional burden of looking after another person in such deep distress is made worse by the fact that so often the carer is a wife, husband, lover, father or mother. Care-givers are also under enormous social, practical, physical and emotional pressure (very often carers themselves are physically unwell). Finally, unlike almost any other mental illness, this is a disease that we all know may await us too at the end of our lives. There is always the thought that 'it could be me'.

All of this makes working with people with dementia uniquely challenging. So how do carers in the home, the hospital and the nursing home cope with the emotional strain that looking after someone with dementia places upon them? One way is to depersonalise the person with dementia. In this way it is possible to avoid having to think about the suffering that would be involved if people with dementia were aware of what was happening to them. The medical model, with its emphasis upon dementia as an illness affecting the brain, can be seen in this light as part of the process of shutting out awareness. The creation of a discrete process, something that happens to some people but not others, serves to distance us from the human tragedy involved in 'losing one's mind'.

In order to cope on an intrapsychic level with the emotional threat of such work, therefore, carers often adopt defences such as denial and depersonalisation, whereby the sufferer is not thought to have 'insight'. Care-giving can come to be treated almost as if it were just a matter of 'common sense'

(Kitwood and Bredin 1992). Placing the memory loss of old age into the organic framework means that those who work with dementia sufferers do not have to be empathic (although many clearly are). The medical model does not require them to place themselves into emotional contact with the suffering of others.

Moreover, given the near-complete lack of supervision to enable staff to discuss how their work is affecting them, we can hardly be surprised if periodically their defence mechanisms are overwhelmed and they become unable to attend fully to the emotional needs of their patients.

When the subjective experiences of people with dementia are ignored dementia sufferers can come to be viewed, significantly, as non-people. Non-people, of course, cannot relate, cannot love, and so on. While we can argue that this view of people with dementia is incorrect, nevertheless it has often been the prevailing view. This, in turn, has a serious effect on the way in which those people who care for dementia sufferers are perceived.

Because the patient has become a non-person, they cannot be in a relationship with their relative(s). The relative is likewise depersonalised into 'a carer'. Rather than seeing the relationship as one which the sufferer and relative are struggling to maintain, this faulty analysis hypothesises a non-relationship – a fault which is then further compounded. The stress of relatives is not seen as normally distributed, and instead carers are split into saints ('I don't know how they manage') and sinners (dealing with a frail old lady abusively or manipulatively). Such stereotypes cannot be helpful.

Seeing dementia sufferers as non-people or as people beyond help has also lead to a focus on the carer as the person in need. In the USA, Cotrell and Schulz (1993) have been highly critical of the previous policy, social research and practice agenda in dementia care, which they saw as focusing exclusively upon family carers, disempowering further people with dementia. We would also question, in this context, why the value-rich and multi-faceted term 'relative' has been replaced by the seemingly objective role of 'carer'.

'Carer' is something of a label that permits unskilled (and therefore cheap) forms of care to develop. Caring is actually not simply a matter of common sense – it is very difficult and challenging. The framing of the relationship between carer and sufferer as a burden prevents the examination of other forms of relationship. For instance, we can learn from the people that we work with, and gain from these relationships.

The prejudices that relate to a given person determine how little they 'deserve' (i.e. the more negative slots they occupy, the less they 'deserve'). It follows that the person with dementia is very undeserving. Indeed, the contemporary debate on euthanasia can be seen, in one light, as questioning whether such people deserve even to live. Of course, the debate is not framed in such terms. Rather, they will be put out of their misery. This is richly ironic. A society which has shown almost no interest in the subjective state or experience of these worthless people now cites this experience as the reason for their lives terminating.

Of more concern to us in the present context is the poor level of services – especially in terms of therapy – available to people with dementia. As we showed in the previous section, they have almost no access to therapy or even counselling. Where there *are* services, they are actually for the relatives of people with dementia rather than the sufferers themselves. Respite care and carers groups are two obvious examples. Day care is often described in terms of 'giving the carers a break' (note again that the relatives have lost their identities as wifes/daughters/sons/husbands and become homogenised into 'carers'). The lack of interest in sufficient stimulation and person-care is all too evident in the weak legislation governing residential and nursing homes.

Thus stereotypes and prejudices are not neutral – they directly support poor services of limited quality and quantity. They aggregate stereotypes, so that a person with dementia is in 'multiple jeopardy', to use Alison Norman's phrase (1985); and as a result, people with dementia are particularly disadvantaged in terms of service delivery. Indeed, many of the limited services that do exist are there not for them but for their carers.

For the relative, being reduced to the role of carer removes at a stroke their relationship with their spouse or parent and its years of history; and, having stripped away all the spoken and unspoken 'there and thens', allows only the 'here and now' of organic brain damage to be considered. The majority of carers with whom we have worked in clinical practice did not see their husbands, wives, fathers and mothers as 'burdens'. Care-giving was stressful, hard and terribly demanding, but they did not want to give it up until they were sure that they could no longer meet their loved one's needs. The relationship and the love continued, albeit in new forms. Moreover, even when the needs of their husbands, wives, fathers or mothers were greatest, these carers rarely saw the act of caring as a one-way street in which they gave but did not receive. The relationships were far more complex than this and could not be described solely in terms of burden and stress.

Overview: The shifting emphasis within dementia care and research

Imagine for a moment that you work with people with dementia, perhaps as a care or nursing assistant. You may have received some formal training on the illness of dementia, and may have a fair idea about what to expect from the sufferers that you work with. You will have been told that by and large, with some small fluctuations, people with dementia become steadily less capable.

Imagine now that you and your colleagues have put in a lot of hard work to raise the quality of life of one particular dementia sufferer (we shall call her Mary) who has recently joined your group. At first the work is hard, and there is little apparent change in the patient. Over time, however, you notice that she begins to do things that you had not seen her do before. Mary begins to smile more often and occasionally makes a funny remark about something that is happening around her. She takes more interest in her appearance and starts to remember your name and those of your colleagues.

Now these changes are wonderful, and you are rightly proud of Mary and what you and she have achieved. But what sense can you make of what has happened? If the only understanding that you have of dementia derives from the organic model, then it will be very hard for you to understand the situation. Perhaps you will be able to explain some of the changes by noting that there have been improvements in Mary's physical condition. Perhaps one of your colleagues will say that no wonder Mary is less depressed now, after all, as people with dementia grow more confused and forget what has happened to them. But we suspect that there will still be much that you will find hard to understand. Put simply, the organic model does not give you a language that you can use to make sense of what you are seeing. The only language that the model gives you is this:

- People with dementia get worse
- If somebody with dementia seems to be getting better then this means they were not ill in the first place.

Consequently, there is a great temptation to set aside that which does not fit in with the medical model, such as evidence which suggests that people with dementia can make better use of their abilities and can improve, if only for a short period of time. This simple medical understanding cannot explain all the evidence.

Thirty years ago, the eminent British psychiatrist, Stengel (1964), wrote:

> What is needed more than another definition (of 'dementia') is a re-examination of the whole concept. Possibly it will be found to be too

broad, too vague, too unsophisticated for our time and be given a place in the museum of psychiatric terms.

By representing symptoms of dementia as purely individual in nature, the standard paradigm model fails to leave any space for either the personal or the social. Yet the social–psychological factors are important. For instance, the emotional and cognitive effects of relocation and the impact of life events (Orrell and Davies 1994) on the well-being of elderly people in general and of people with dementia more specifically (Orrell and Bebbington 1993) are important experiences that shape people's lives. Yet with respect to institutionalisation, for example, two recent texts reviewing, respectively, linguistic and neuropsychological research on the elderly (Maxim and Bryan 1994; Hart and Semple 1994), both with copious pages of references, do not devote a single line to the possible effects of institutionalisation on linguistic and cognitive performance.

More generally, the importance of paying attention to the social–psychological environment surrounding older people has been increasingly recognised. Thus social gerontologists have stressed the detrimental impact that social stereotypes of ageing have upon older people (e.g. Hockey and James 1993; Bytheway 1995). Coupland, Nussbaum and Coupland 1991, for example, have reviewed the literature on intergenerational talk and suggest that the speech of younger people changes when they are addressing older people so that the older person feels that they are being put in a position where they have to disclose painful information about themselves. The authors suggest that the contrasting expectations and role-stereotypes of older and younger people place the former in a position whereby miscommunication is likely, if not inevitable.

Where the older person has been diagnosed as suffering from a dementing process other social factors are also important. For instance, Kitwood and Bredin (1992) have argued powerfully that once someone has been diagnosed as having a progressive memory loss they are subjected to a debilitating onslaught both from within and from the outside world. Similarly, Hockey and James (1993) have stressed how the metaphors frequently used to describe elderly people with dementia link ageing to helplessness and dependency (e.g. the phrase 'he/she is experiencing a second childhood'). The concept of the interaction between psychosocial factors and neurological impairment is hardly new. Rothschild (1937; 1942; Rothschild and Sharp 1941) invoked this relationship to explain the discrepancies he observed between clinical and pathological severity (Hart and Semple 1994, p.44). Kahn (1965) originated the term 'excess disability' to highlight the discrepancy which exists when the individual's functional incapacity is greater than that warranted by the actual impairment (Brody *et al.* 1971, p.125). Brody *et al.* designed treatment programmes for mentally impaired elderly patients aimed at combating these excess disabilities.

In the last few years, considerable research interest has focused on the link between education and occupation and both Alzheimer's disease and vascular forms of dementia. A number of studies in the United States have found an association between higher levels of education and types of occupation (involving greater interpersonal skills or physical demands) and a lower risk of dementia (e.g. Mortimer and Graves 1993; Mortel *et al.* 1994). Similar findings have been reported in Italy (Bonaiuto *et al.* 1995), Holland (Ott *et al.* 1995) and Spain (Bartolome and Fernandez 1995). This remains a controversial area: some studies do not report a link at all (Beard *et al.* 1992), others find that later age of onset and a greater level of symptom severity is associated with less education (Moritz and Petitti 1993), while others suggest that occupation is an independent risk factor even when education is controlled for (Stern *et al.* 1995).

Although we do not wish to dwell too long on this point, we have been struck by the way in which this relationship is accounted for in terms of education and occupation providing a 'reserve' that counters the effects of dementia, or in terms of 'lifelong mental stimulation and neuronal growth' (Stern *et al.* 1995). A comprehensive explanation is missing. It is simply not good enough to provide an explanation for one set of factors (the importance of education, occupation and social class) through a model which refers exclusively to the operation of causes at another level. It is as if we only had models of bereavement which accounted for grief reactions solely in terms of a deficit or excess of certain neurotransmitters. The establishment of a relationship between psychosocial factors and dementia only serves to draw attention to the absence of a psychosocial framework within which to place these findings.

In the rest of this book we will show how the traditional psychiatric diagnostic system can only be part of the study of dementia, and how a broader psychological understanding has developed. We do not, however, wish to deny that the research using this paradigm has considerable validity and utility. Our argument is that an exclusive reliance on this model has caused data and research that have not fitted into the model to be ignored or minimised. It is not that the organic model of dementia is right and that others are wrong, or vice-versa: it is just that the exclusive reliance on the organic model at the expense of others has tended to limit the sorts of care that have been available.

The standard paradigm of dementia care, we have argued, has little room for psychological and social factors. But it does not have to be this way. It is possible to have a dialogue between the psychological and psychiatric approaches and blend social and biochemical research together so that clinical practice becomes more effective.

Summary of main points

- Until recently, the organic disease model of dementia could be said to have had paradigmatic status. That is to say there was near-uniform agreement that within this model lay the complete explanation of dementia. This monolithic approach has had quite severe consequences in terms of excluding other perspectives and considerations.

- The process of making a diagnosis of dementia is a difficult one, and relies too heavily on the unfounded assumption that there is a straightforward link between neurological damage, cognitive change and symptomatic behaviour.

- There is a large literature on disability, mainly in relation to physical handicaps. The disability model has the merit of specifying what is actually missing/damaged rather than simply describing a disease that eats into all abilities and personhood. Therefore, a disability model could specify more exactly how a person with dementia could be helped and how their environment could be more user-friendly.

- People with dementia experience the changes within their internal world within the context of a lifetime of experiences. We can only understand their reactions to this process if we can understand how they have been affected by and dealt with past traumas and other formative events.

- The organic model's emphasis upon brain functioning and cognitive loss has meant that those people who care for dementia sufferers have tended to be seen within a simplified role. But a carer's relationship with their husband, wife, father or mother is invariably a complex one, and often one in which both parties are able to give as well as to receive.

- People with dementia tend to be seen as existing outside a social world, with all their problems attributed to brain damage and with the effects of the social world in which they live too often discounted. One of the major changes of recent years is that this partial view has been challenged and a new body of work has emerged which emphasises the importance of basing dementia care around the personhood of the dementia sufferer.

- Emotions and emotional states are seen in the organic model as 'symptoms' deriving from neurological damage. They have no independent validity as the reactions of people terrified by what is happening to them.

- The experiences of people with dementia are frequently neglected, yet to believe you are losing your mind must be terrifying.

CHAPTER 5

Therapeutic Disdain

Therapy, Therapists and People with Dementia

In this chapter we shall look at the lack of psychotherapy for people with dementia in particular and for older people generally; at how this arose; and at the various therapeutic methods that were developed during and after the 1980s for people with dementia.

It will be clear by now that the standard paradigm or model of dementia takes little account of what the patient feels or thinks. The impetus of the biomedical model of dementia is towards finding genetic and chemical cures for dementia. Although there may well be clear benefits from this kind of work there are also potential dangers, for instance from toxic reactions, the possibility of over-prescribing, and poor reactions to drugs such as minor and especially major (anti-psychotic) tranquillisers (McGrath and Jackson 1996; McShane *et al.* 1997).

In this vacuum it might be thought that psychotherapists and counsellors would want to offer people with dementia therapy or counselling, as obviously the condition is highly distressing. In fact, there is very little such therapy available to people with dementia. Apparently it is not seen as useful or likely to be effective. So there is no range of alternative ideas and treatments offered by therapists to counter the organic model. It is not as if there was a contest that psychotherapy lost – it never attempted to compete. So the standard paradigm gets yet more credibility and credence by being the *only* explanation.

It is important to understand that people with dementia are not denied psychotherapy because memory difficulties make the process difficult. This might have some validity, as we shall discuss at length in later chapters. But the reason why they are offered no psychotherapy is that they are old.

We will try to explain how this situation arose. Effectively, psychotherapy started with the work of Sigmund Freud and Josef Breuer in Vienna at the end of the last century (Breuer and Freud 1955; First published 1895). Freud went on to develop the first theory or school of therapy – psychoanalysis. In 1904 he gave a paper in which he suggested various limitations to his new method of psychoanalysis (Freud 1953; First published 1905). Among these were 'those patients who do not possess a reasonable degree of education and a fairly reliable character' (p.263). In the same paper, he also wrote that:

> near or above the age of fifty the elasticity of the mental processes, on which the treatment depends, is as a rule lacking – old people are no longer educable – and, on the other hand, the mass of material to be dealt with would prolong the duration of the treatment indefinitely. (p.264)

What his followers did with such an early and tentative paper is interesting. In the case of the elderly:

> sadly, what was only a rule of thumb for an emerging psychotherapist became a rigid operating rule and in Great Britain the official institution governing psychoanalysis, the British Psychoanalytic Society has until this year refused to accept patients over the age of 40. (Hildebrand 1986, p.23)

The simplest explanation appears to be that psychoanalysts framed rules of exclusion to remove the less attractive of those needing help with little or no respect for the evidence relating to those exclusions. The illogicality of using Freud's 1904 paper as the basis for therapeutic decisions is shown by a later paper of his. Returning to the theme of untreatability in a lecture in 1916, this time in relation to psychosis, he writes:

> [Psychoanalysis] is as powerless [for the time being at least] against these ailments as any other form of therapy ... Will you be inclined to maintain on that account that an analysis of such cases is to be rejected because it is fruitless? I think not. We have a right, or rather a duty, to carry on our research without consideration of any immediate beneficial effect. (Freud 1955, p.235)

It is clear, then, that in 1904 Freud was summarising some rules of thumb from his clinical experience, not expressing any strong convictions. His followers took these dicta as law because it suited them.

There never was any particular logic to Freud's argument. Thus the eminent psychotherapist Robert Butler has argued the opposite – that older people make excellent candidates for psychotherapy as they are in a hurry: 'probably at no other time in life is there as potent a force toward self-awareness operating as in old age' (Butler 1963). The important underlying variables are economics and client attractiveness. Psychotherapy and the various schools of psychoanalysis are highly verbal techniques and so require patients who are verbally fluent; and because most psychotherapy is private and expensive, it also requires people who are working. This economic necessity seems to have been turned perversely into an ageist stance.

The question of the purpose of working with someone with a poor memory can only be answered by looking at what 'being therapeutic' means. Unfortunately, people confuse the *technique* of therapy with the *purpose*. The technique of therapy is most usually a one-hour talk session, which would not be very suitable for people with dementia, especially if it is advanced. But there is no reason to accept that this is the only way to do 'therapy'.

It may be argued that therapy is about assessing the problem, treating it and hopefully curing it. You cannot apply the assess–treat–cure model, which is borrowed from medicine, to dementia, because you cannot cure dementia. But again this is to accept a limited view of what 'therapy' is. We want to suggest that the purpose of therapy is to improve people's sense of well-being; to increase the resources they have available to relate to their physical and interpersonal world; and to improve their quality of life.

You can see that these goals make no mention of 'talking cures'. They do not specify how the goals should be achieved, because there are many techniques, as we hope to show you in the later chapters. So if 'therapy' is about maintaining quality of life and does not only mean talking, it follows that it may well not be necessary for the person to have a good memory in order to benefit from our therapeutic work.

Nor would less verbal approaches expect a 'cure'. But the whole idea of 'cures' in mental health is a curious one. Throughout our lives we will hit crises and go through good and bad times. So periodically we are likely to need help – be it from friends or from professionals – to sort out what we are feeling and what we should do. Staying mentally well is an ongoing process, not a once-and-for-all state.

Each school of psychotherapy teaches only one approach, be it Jungian or Rogerian or whatever. But one thing we hope you will get out of this book is an idea of the importance of flexibility. Those working with people with dementia will need to change their style with each individual, depending on their interests, needs and abilities.

Psychotherapists who train for many years and at considerable personal expense naturally want the world to believe that theirs is the most skilled and difficult work. This is baloney. They are working with highly verbal, highly intelligent people who often just need to slow down and make some time and space to sort themselves out.

Those who work with people with dementia are often working with very damaged people, who are also trying to make sense of their world but finding it terribly difficult because their skills of understanding and interacting with the world have been diminished. With dementia, it is the worker who has to create the conditions in which people can feel secure and relate. If these conditions are not provided, then the person with dementia just will not be able to make the progress that they need to make.

In the 1980s interest in working with older people increased among clinical psychologists. Individual therapy with cognitively capable older people was undertaken and written up by a number of authors (Sherman 1981; Hildebrand 1986; Knight 1986; 1992) so the unwillingness to even see older adults in therapy became less pronounced. A number of types of therapy were put forward. These included Reality Orientation (Holden and Woods 1995; First published 1982); Reminiscence (Norris and Abu El Eileh 1982; Norris 1986); Validation (Feil 1990; First published 1982) and Kitwood's work on reversing the malignant social psychology of the institution (1997b).

There are three points of interest to comment on about these methods. First, none came out of the main psychotherapy schools – Freud, Jung, Berne etc. – so they do not represent a change of heart or of focus among the major therapy schools. Second, they tend to utilise groupwork rather than individual work. However, it is individual work that is considered most efficacious and certainly most prestigious in our society. We can see how money and prestige define the quality of service by comparing a privately-bought hour of psychoanalysis with a service in the public domain such as a social work group for carers (Table 5.1).

Third, all these methods are focused on the institutionalised person. Reality Orientation and Reminiscence are concerned with the person in a residential unit. The staff are exhorted to set up a Reality Orientation classroom or run Reminiscence groups. Validation and Kitwood's work are more concerned with the more severe dementia to be found in nursing homes or hospital wards.

Table 5.1 Comparisons of prestige symbols in two settings	
Private (Psychoanalytic session)	*Public (Social work group)*
Buying	Being given/charity
Exclusive use of therapist	Sharing less prestigiously qualified leader
Uninterrupted time	Possibility of the session being interrupted by telephone calls, other clients and unexpected crises
In prestige setting	When was group room last painted? Most likely 'down town'
Will focus on concerns of living well in the metropolis	Will focus on surviving
Will aggregate to a large amount of time	Time available will be limited; group may be terminated by lack of resources rather than client wishes

The point is not that these interventions are not useful, although empirical support has not been clear-cut (Thorton and Brotchie 1987; Holden and Woods 1995; Woods 1996). Rather, it is that most people with dementia live in their own homes in the community (Gordon and Spicker 1997). So one message implicit in these important therapies is actually rather negative – namely, that most old people with dementia are institutionalised (Bender 1998). The reality is, of course, that it is most *psychologists* writing about dementia care who are institution-based.

To complete the picture, the 1980s saw the rise of Cognitive-Behaviour Therapy (Beck 1976; Dick, Gallagher-Thompson and Thompson 1996). This very rapidly expanding set of ideas was applied to anxiety and depression, relatively independently of age. Thus, Yost *et al.* (1986) developed a group cognitive therapy model for depressed older adults. Similarly, since the early 1990s there have been small-scale attempts to apply psychodynamic ideas to dementia (e.g. Sinason 1992).

We shall look at the ideas of these writers in much greater detail in Part Two. However, these are individual and isolated initiatives. The basic lack of interest and practical concern among psychotherapists remains. There are still few publicly-available psychotherapy services for older people and none for people with dementia.

Summary of major points

- The location of the psychotherapy schools in the private sector led to a need for potential patients to be verbal, well-heeled and, given the long periods of interaction between therapist and patient, attractive to work with. By 1904, Freud had excluded the over-fifties. Whether he meant this exclusion as an absolute rule or as a guideline is open to debate.

- The marginal position of the older adults in our population has meant that psychotherapy services for their age group, as opposed to those for children or young adults, are underdeveloped. As a very non-prestigious subgroup, people with dementia attracted even less interest. The therapy system, through lack of interest, has left people with dementia to professionals utilising the organic model, and thereby strengthened this model further by providing no alternative.

- If the condition is regarded as irreversible then attempts to provide therapy, especially psychotherapy, must be a waste of time and resources. One direct effect of therapeutic nihilism is the very high use of untrained staff found in the field of dementia care. This is hardly surprising if sophisticated efforts requiring trained staff are regarded as a waste of time.

- This nihilism also makes it hard to arouse practitioner interest in developing and researching new methods of psychological intervention. Because of the therapeutic nihilism there is little belief that these could be useful and little money or professional encouragement made available for their development.

- In their work with the adult well-heeled, psychotherapists profess great respect and concern for the needs and well-being of their clients. But through their complete lack of interest and ageism, psychotherapists of the various schools implicitly see people with dementia as lower status – devalued people to be looked after by devalued staff.

Overview of Part One

As you reach the end of Part One, we hope we have given you a good introduction to the current model of dementia; its historical development; the lack of competing explanations; and some of its weaknesses. We will look at the economic and professional factors maintaining the model in Chapters 15 and 16.

We now want to look at an alternative understanding of what is happening to a person who is experiencing cognitive difficulties.

Constructing a Psychological Model of Dementia

CHAPTER 6

Introducing the Person-focused Approach
What is it Like to be a Person Diagnosed as Having Dementia?

> In the majority of research on AD, the afflicted person is viewed as a disease entity to be studied rather than someone who can contribute to our understanding of the illness and its course. By not exploring the individual's experience of the disease, we may have overlooked a source for understanding some of the immense variability in the presentation and progression of the illness. (Cotrell and Schulz 1993, p.205)

In Part Two of this book we want to try to see the world through the eyes of someone who has been told, or someone who perhaps just suspects, that they have dementia. Our focus is on the person with dementia and on how the changes that are involved in this illness affect their thinking and feelings. The orientation of this book is therefore a *person-focused* one (Bender 1996a; Bender and Cheston 1997), and it is this person-focused approach that we will outline in this chapter.

Imagine that this morning you could not remember the name of a friend. You probably wouldn't worry unduly – after all, slips of the memory like this are pretty common and we understand that they can be caused by many different factors. Perhaps you have been overworking recently, or perhaps, you think, 'it's just one of those things'. But now imagine that you are 75 years old and it has been on your mind recently that you might be starting to dement. This otherwise insignificant memory lapse could, for such a person, represent yet another piece of evidence that they are going down the road to institutionalisation and incontinence. It would be terrifying, wouldn't it? So we can see the importance of the construction or frame that a person places on a given event.

In fact, the situation is even more complicated. The person's relatives and friends may also note the small lapses in memory and other strange behaviours and construe them as indicating that something is wrong. They, in turn, may experience fear, panic and dismay – and their reaction will, in turn, impact upon the person.

Ultimately, the concerns of the person and those around them may lead to the arrival of one of those in society to whom we have been taught to turn at times of need – in this case a doctor, psychiatrist, nurse or psychologist. The *act of diagnosis* of dementia, when it arrives, may have a devastating effect on the person, their family and the relationships between the person and their family (Drayton 1995). The interplay between the person and their relatives in terms of what they feel and how they communicate it becomes very complex, and can lead to a further downward spiral in the person's feelings of security within their personal and interpersonal world.

These strong reactions may well be at least as important, and in some cases, more important in determining the person's behaviour than the actual memory loss.

So, the central task for health and social service professionals, as well as for all other carers, is *not* to try to guess which bits of the brain have become damaged. Rather, the central task should be to *understand the subjective world of the person who believes they may have dementia.* This is a *person-focused* approach because it assumes that the most important thing is to understand how that person sees what is happening to them, and not just to look at their brain and how it is functioning. This is the prime meaning of focusing on the person.

But this approach carries with it another important meaning. As we shift our focus towards the needs of the person, so the needs of the care-givers alter within this framework. A person-focused approach implies that we should see care-givers as husbands, wives, sons and daughters. Their needs, both personal and professional, must not be considered in isolation but as part of a couple or family.

Note that we are in no way denying or minimising the distress and heartache felt by relatives who believe that their loved one is 'gone for ever'. All these feelings are strong and real. What we are saying is that to focus solely on that distress is effectively to give up: to accept therapeutic nihilism. To focus on the person with the condition is to hold on to and to bear witness to their struggle to survive amidst the wreckage created by this illness.

A further major aspect is that we have to see beyond the person
dementia and their close circle. To understand how people respond t
problems created by dementia and *the ways open to them to respond*, we neea to
see the person in their cultural and societal context.

The person-focused approach assumes that a person with dementia is a
person trying, as are we all, to make sense of the world they inhabit. Table 6.1
summarises these points.

Table 6.1 The main meanings of 'person-focus' in the understanding of dementia

Focus:

1. on the person with dementia, not their diseased brain

2. on their emotions and understandings, not memory losses

3. on the person within the context of a marriage or a family

4. within a wider society and its values.

We call this approach *person-focused* rather than, for instance, 'person-centred'
(Kitwood 1997b) because we are trying to capture in the term 'focused'
something of that feeling you get when you fiddle with the lens of your
camera and the leaves of that tree, the lines on that rock, come into sharp
focus. At present, because the person with dementia is perceived as a
non-person, we know little about them and see them only vaguely. We are
experts about strangers. Moreover, the term 'person-centred' has resonances
of 'client- centred', a term that is widely used in counselling and which,
although important to the interventions that we will describe later on, has,
nevertheless, a somewhat different purpose.

Let us now try to be a little more specific about the attributes of the
person-focused approach (Table 6.2).

Table 6.2 Features of the person-focused approach to dementia

1. Dementia needs to be understood as an interaction between psychosocial and neurological influences.

2. The main focus of dementia care must be on the person living with the illness, alongside an awareness of the needs of carers.

3. Dementia is a terrifying ordeal which creates an enormous sense of insecurity within individuals and generates an emotional reaction.

4. The impact of the process of dementia is also experienced in terms of a threat to the person's view of themselves as a coherent entity.

5. The threat to a person's identity that is posed by dementia precipitates a range of behaviours whose function is to assert the individual's identity.

6. In order to understand the behaviour of a person living with dementia we also need to understand their fears and the way in which they assert their own identity.

7. Without such an understanding of the emotional and identity needs of dementia sufferers we are liable to misinterpret the behaviour that arises when these needs are not met as resulting from neurological damage.

8. We need to understand how a person with dementia is valued in their society, and the effects – economic and social – of that valuation.

9. Once we have begun to understand the emotional, identity and social frameworks within which a dementia sufferer lives, then we can begin to develop effective, life-enhancing forms of help.

A clinician trying to understand emotional distress will seek an understanding of three aspects of the person's life:

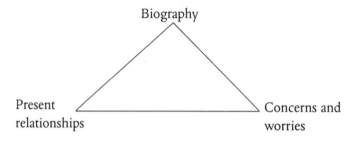

Figure 6.1 The context of emotional distress

1. Their life history, its major events, its crises and how it has formed the person.

2. Their present concerns and worries.

3. Their present network of relationships.

What we are saying is that all these factors will be affecting the thoughts, feelings and behaviour of a person diagnosed as having dementia. At one level – once you have stopped seeing dementia as totally unique and unlike any other form of distress – it is startlingly obvious that these areas should be investigated and understood.

While the core of this approach is to try to understand the individual's subjective experiences, it is important to recognise that these occur within a social context, and therefore we also need to look at the systems that impact on the person with dementia. So it is with the social and ecological world of the dementia sufferer that we will begin our discussion of the person-focused approach in the next chapter. After this we will focus on the subjective experiences of people with dementia and how they cope with what is happening to them.

The second part of this book, then, will attempt to flesh out this brief description of the person-focused approach. In the third part we will draw out the implications of this approach by outlining those patterns of care and forms of psychological intervention that we believe will enhance the ability of the person with dementia to cope with this process of loss and change.

CHAPTER 7

The Person in Context

The Role of Psychological and Social Factors in Dementia

In the first part of the book we presented an overview of current scientific and medical thinking about dementia which accords with the organic model of dementia – what Tom Kitwood has referred to as 'the standard paradigm'. We also outlined some of the criticisms that Kitwood and others have made of this approach. One of the chief criticisms of much of this standard approach is that it does not take sufficient account of the presence of psychological and social factors in the illness.

In this chapter we will develop this argument. We are *not* saying that organic changes do not occur in the brain; and we are *not* saying that these organic changes do not occur independently of any psychological factors; but we *are* saying that we think it very likely that psychological factors *do* contribute to the development of the conditions referred to as 'dementia'. Table 7.1 summarises the main points.

What, then, do we know of the role of psychological and social factors in the development of dementia?

Table 7.1 The main social determinants of the behaviour and feelings of a person with dementia

1. Relatively little behavioural output of a person diagnosed as having dementia is due to the dementia/dementing process.

2. The person diagnosed as having dementia is subjected to a number of negative stereotypes, only one of which is that they are chronically ill. Other important ones are that they are old, ugly, economically useless and resource-wasting.

3. These negative stereotypes are internalised by the person with dementia, leading to beliefs and feelings of uselessness and low mood. Such beliefs and feelings lead to a decreased level of functioning.

4. These negative stereotypes contribute to and are congruent with services of limited quantity and quality available to the person with dementia.

5. Services for people with dementia are non-individual, as individualised service is a high-cost, high-prestige type of service delivery. In contrast, the services for people with dementia are often institutionalised, creating a whole set of very deleterious effects, quite independent from the effects of any brain changes.

Age and ageism

As we described in Part One, there is little diagnosed dementia before the age of 65. Thereafter it increases linearly with age (Ineichen 1987). So, dementia is something that happens almost entirely to older people. To understand dementia, then, we need to understand something of the psychological and social effects of growing old and in particular, we believe, the effects of ageism.

Box 7.1 Ageism

W. Bytheway, in his readable *Ageism* (1995), states:

(a) Ageism generates and reinforces a fear and denigration of the ageing process, and stereotyping presumptions regarding competence and the need for protection.

(b) In particular, ageism legitimates the use of chronological age to mark out classes of people who are systematically denied resources and opportunities that others enjoy, and who suffer the consequences of such denigration, ranging from well-meaning patronage to unambigious vilification. (p.14)

We live in a society that places great emphasis on age. The younger you are, it appears, the better. While so called 'youthful' qualities are respected and valued, the process of growing old is, by comparison, often mocked or derided. One part of this process of devaluing old age is the relatively common attitude that old age is *inevitably* a time of decline involving mental and physical ill-health and marked by poverty and a poor environment. Such views can lead to a process of stereotyping, whereby the expectations of others are affected, leading to a self-fulfilling hypothesis.

This is not to say that ageing does not involve many changes that occur *gradually* as individuals grow older. However, some of these changes occur only after the age of 75–80, while others are a result of the ageing process as a whole (which starts far earlier) rather than being specific to old age. Often, partly as a consequence of ageist stereotypes, those changes that do occur are misinterpreted as the unavoidable consequences of ageing. In fact, there are many things that we can do to improve the quality of an individual's life.

Ageism, or the holding of negative social stereotypes about older people and the process of ageing, has been well investigated over the last decade and more (e.g. Rowe 1994; Bytheway 1995). Not only are there contemporary societal prejudices such as the lack of equal opportunities in applying for jobs, but the valuing of youth over age also takes subtler forms, from the images of the ideal man or woman as young (in their twenties), thin and with smooth skin to be seen in almost any colour magazine, to the representation of older people as non-productive. Indeed, hostility to non-workers is perhaps the key prejudice as it routinely affects all retired people.

There is, therefore, a tendency within our society to represent old age as a time of idleness and increasing illness, and elderly people as having nothing to contribute and being an economic, if not psychological, burden to society, wasting huge amounts of scarce resources and valuable time.

The effects of these stereotypes can be seen in two ways. First of all, they may have a direct effect on the lives of older people by changing the way in which those around them behave towards them. Giles (1991) for instance, has shown that young care-givers in nursing homes wrongly assume that the elderly residents they care for will want to talk about themselves. The conversation is therefore set up by the care-givers in such a way that residents feel pressured into disclosing personal information about themselves.

However, a much larger effect of stereotypes is that they can be *internalised*. Internalisation, in this context, means taking in negative social stereotypes about elderly people and believing them to be true about oneself.

So, if you are considered by society as valueless, internalisation is seeing yourself as useless.

As a result of both this internalisation and the altered behaviour of other people, levels of self-esteem can drop and the person's mood can become lowered. Thus the negative stereotypes involved in ageing can lead to low mood, decreased motivation and reduced opportunities to take part in social activities. The trouble with this (besides being a rather miserable and unenjoyable way of living) is that it can have a knock-on effect on the person's ability to remember information and thus contribute to the diagnosis of dementia and its (apparent) severity. Figure 7.1 illustrates this vicious spiral.

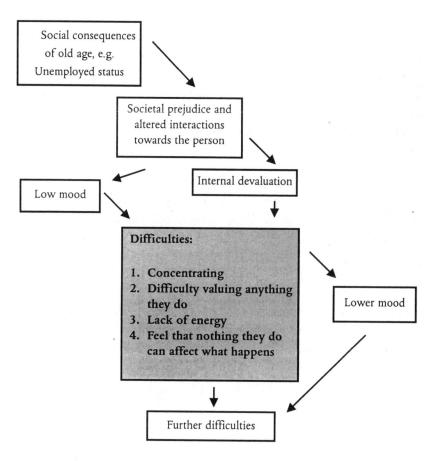

Figure 7.1 Vicious spiral following the internalisation of societal devaluation of unemployed status
Source : Adapted from Bender, Bauckham and Norris (1999)

Empirical evidence for the debilitating effects of ageism has been provided by Rodin and Langer (1980), while Levy and Langer (1994) have produced strong evidence to link the acceptance of negative stereotypes to increased memory loss. This pattern of internalised devaluation is of importance to all those who work with older people, including those who work with people with dementia:

1. We have to acknowledge that an old person may see little reason to improve their self-image. But we need to aim at improving self-image and self-esteem since, if we can, we will improve that part of the memory which is decreased by the depressed mood.

2. More generally, we need to work on mood, because depressed people find that even the simplest act – like making a cup of tea – takes ages and requires a huge amount of energy.

A particularly effective way of reversing the internalisation of devaluation is by helping people to talk with each other in a group setting. Not only is the person valued by the group leaders but also by their peers. While we cannot do much about what society does to our clients, we can at least attempt to affect their internalisation of this devaluation.

Gender differences

Women are more at risk of developing dementia than men. Many surveys (e.g. Gordon and Spicker 1997) give rates per 1000 population for older people. These rates will always show an excess of women due to differential mortality. However, there are a number of studies which do give data *within* each sex.

The Guy's/Age Concern Survey (Lindesay, Briggs and Murphy 1989) sampled 890 people aged 65+ in Lewisham and North Southwark Health District. The measure of interest to us was the Organic Brain Syndrome and Depression Scale of the Comprehensive Assessment and Referral Evaluation (CARE) Schedule (Gurland *et al.* 1983; First published 1977), which was used as a measure of dementia. Table 7.2 below gives the results.

Severity Range	OBS Score	Men (%)	Women (%)
Mild–Severe	3+	3.9	5.1
Moderate–Severe	4+	2.0	3.9
Severe Only	6+	0.8	1.3

Table 7.2 The Guy's/Age Concern Survey – Rates of dementia

Source: Lindesay, Briggs and Murphy (1989) p.320

It can be seen that whatever range is chosen, women are in each case more at risk than are men.

Morgan *et al.* (1992), using the Clifton Assessment Procedures for the Elderly (CAPE) (Pattie and Gilleard 1975) and a clinical interview, report an incidence across four years in their Nottingham study of 2.9 per cent for men and 5.2 per cent for women. Finally, Hagnell, Ojesso and Rorsman (1992) report, in their survey of Lundby in Sweden, that the lifetime risks of contracting DAT were 25.5 per cent for men and 31.9 per cent for women. The multi-infarct figures are 29.8 per cent for men and 25.1 per cent for women; but since this is the less frequent subdiagnosis, it does not affect the validity of our overall conclusion: women are more susceptible to dementia than men.

Clearly there are many possible differences, both biological and social, that may account for these findings. One significant difference that has been implicated in other gender-based research in mental health concerns the differential loss of social role. This has at least three implications. First, because of differential rates of mortality, men are less likely to lose their spouse and the presence of a spouse – following Brown and Harris (1978) and Murphy (1982) – is likely to be a buffer factor against a variety of stressors.

Second, the role of widower is arguably more acceptable and flexible than the role of widow. As there are fewer widowers, their presence among a group of widows can attract more interest and support and thus offer a higher social value than the more frequent role of widow.

Finally, there is evidence that men tend to have a wider range of social roles available to them, and that these are accorded higher status. The loss of one role, for instance due to retirement, can therefore be more easily compensated for by developing the remaining roles. We will return to the issue of role loss later on in this section.

Occupation, social class and education

As we described in Chapter 4, there is considerable evidence of an association between a (higher) level of education and a (lower) level of dementia, e.g. in America, Mortimer and Graves (1993) and Mortel *et al.* (1994); in Italy, Bonaiuto *et al.* (1995); in Holland, Ott *et al.* (1995); and in Spain, Bartolome and Fernandez (1995).

Consistently significant correlations have also been found between dementia and social class. For example, Lindesay, Briggs and Murphy (1989), in a large survey of Lewisham and North Southwark, already mentioned, report an overall rate of 4.6 per cent for cognitive impairment. Cognitive impairment is taken as scoring as three or higher on the Organic Brain Syndrome of Gurland *et al.*'s CARE Schedule (1983). Broken down by social class, the rates are:

Table 7.3 The Guy's/Age Concern Survey – rates of dementia by social class	
Social Class	*Rate*
I/II	0%
III non-manual	1.3%
III manual	4.0%
IV/V	7.3%

Malignant social psychology

People with dementia often receive institutional care, be it within health/social service establishments or private residential or nursing homes. Goffman (1961), in his well known and influential book *Asylums*, highlighted the characteristics of such institutions – their degradation and de-individualising of the person through block treatment etc. Goffman was providing a sociological perspective. The psychiatrist Russell Barton (1976; First published 1959), in a rather drier style, outlined the resultant individual behaviour as 'institutional neurosis'. These very strong environmental controls of behaviour will demand and elicit certain types of behaviour, quite independent of diagnosis or brain condition. Indeed, 'institutionalisation' was developed as a concept to explain the behaviour of long-stay patients such as chronic schizophrenics (cf. Wing and Brown 1970).

These ideas first had practical implications in the field of learning disability. Wolf Wolfensberger (1972; 1975), with his concept of normal-isation, launched a concerted attack against dehumanising practices (Brown and Smith 1992). The thrust of normalisation, later renamed Social Role Valorisation, was that all people, regardless of level of ability, should be treated as having equal value and should have access to valued social roles and all the elements of a normal life. The King's Fund (1985) have adapted these principles to the area of dementia care and have suggested that the services available to older adults should follow the basic principles set down by normalisation.

More recently, Tom Kitwood has applied a somewhat similar social psychological focus to the field of dementia. In a series of papers, brought together in his book *Dementia Reconsidered* (1997b), he has highlighted such negative and deleterious treatment of human beings by more powerful others in his concept of a 'malignant social psychology'.

Tom Kitwood argues that the losses involved in dementia concern not only the loss of neurological functioning but also involve a change in the dementia sufferer's relationships with other people. For people who are subsequently given the label of 'Alzheimer's disease' or another form of dementia, this process begins with the individual's behaviour being interpreted as in some way different from the norm. As we have described above, from this point onwards, their behaviour and talk is likely to be interpreted in terms of the cognitive deficits of the individual.

Kitwood goes on to argue that a *malignant social psychology* (MSP) surrounds people once they have been diagnosed as having a progressive memory loss. Consequently, people with dementia are subjected to a debilitating onslaught both from within and from the outside world. He has described a number of different ways in which the social world in which a dementia sufferer lives and is cared for can combine with the neurological impairment to erode their sense of being – their personhood, as he has defined it. For instance, they can be *disempowered* (things are done for them that they are able to do for themselves), *infantilised* (by being treated as if they had returned to a childhood state) and *intimidated* (for instance by psychologists and others asking them apparently irrelevant questions as part of their assessment of memory functioning) (*see also* Chapters 12 and 14).

Kitwood draws on the work of the philosopher Martin Buber (1958) and sees personhood as arising from a human being's interaction with others. Personhood is essentially social: it refers to human beings in relation to others. But it also carries ethical considerations: to be a person is to have a certain status and to be worthy of respect (Kitwood and Bredin 1992).

Given the representation of dementia as involving losses in both the social and the neurological domains, Kitwood has developed a way of intervening within social (and in particular institutional) environments. The psychosocial quality of the care that surrounds an individual can be assessed through the process of Dementia Care Mapping, helping ward and nursing home staff to identify those aspects of their care practices that are demeaning or devaluing and contrast these with those aspects that help to preserve personhood. It attempts to create a culture within which significant changes in the social psychology surrounding dementia sufferers can occur. These changes leave open the possibility that *rementia* – positive changes in the dementia sufferer's functioning – can occur. We will describe this process in more detail in later chapters.

Tom Kitwood has been an inspirational force for change within dementia care. Without his work it is hard to see how the 'new culture of dementia care' could have existed in anything like the form that it currently does. He has emphasised the importance of a person-centred form of care, and of seeing the *person* with dementia rather than the person with *dementia* – themes that we have emphasised in this book. However, the impact of Kitwood's ideas has, until recently, been largely confined to the culture of care within institutions such as nursing homes and wards. There is also a need to address the ways in which individuals with dementia and their relatives can be helped to develop effective and sustainable patterns of interaction within their own homes. Waiting to intervene until the person with dementia is confined to an institution is leaving matters rather late.

The interaction between organic and social-psychological factors

The existence of these social and psychological factors has, indeed, been known for some time, and is largely uncontroversial. However, many of the standard paradigm accounts see the primary cause as lying in genetic, molecular and organic changes.

The (negative) relationship of dementia and education has been explained in terms of education providing a 'reserve' to counter the effects of dementia by providing more neuronal growth (Stern *et al.* 1995), but this is obviously an incomplete explanation. It explains behaviour at one level as if it could have the same meaning at another level. 'Being in love' is not the same as excitation of neurones in a given part of your brain; education, in itself, does not cause neuronal growth.

Instead we feel that there is likely to be a much more complex and subtle interaction between organic and psychosocial factors than most researchers and clinicians working within the standard paradigm currently seem prepared to admit to. Indeed, we feel that there is strong reason to believe that psychological and social factors can have some influence, if not on the rate of neurological change, then at the very least on the ability of the individual to withstand neurological damage.

Social roles and dementia

One way to bring together these apparently disparate groups of psychological risk factors is to consider them in terms of a common, unifying factor – that of the loss of social roles. By role, we mean those aspects of a person's affect, meaning and behaviour systems with which they structure their interpersonal world. Individuals in a given society occupy a wide range of roles which support their definitions of self. Common major roles would include those of worker, wage earner, husband or wife, parent, member of an organisation such as a club or a hobby/activity group, etc. Most roles utilised by older people will have positive social valuations attached to them. Therefore, the loss of any role will result in decreased social valuation or prestige.

The precipitant of major role loss is *not* age. Rather, the precipitants are the age-related factors of: (a) increased infirmity (and energy loss); (b) decreased mobility; and (c) loss of network of effectively important others (Wenger 1994a), and of close others, for example through the death of a spouse. Thus the risk of dementia developing in a given individual is proportional to: (a) the loss of the capacity to fulfil roles (health and mobility); (b) the presence/loss of important others; and (c) decreased motivation to interact through lowered mood or grieving (see Figure 7.2).

We know that the availability of valued social roles often decreases with age. We also know that, in broad terms, the higher the social position and the greater the level of education that a person has completed, the more roles they are likely to have available to them. Moreover, the network of these roles is more likely to be subtle and varied, and the social roles are likely to be more highly valued. A similar pattern can often be found for men and women but the social roles available to women tend to be fewer and to be more tightly circumscribed.

The importance of having a broad, highly-valued network of social roles can be seen when something happens to disrupt the person's life. This is often referred to as a *life event* (Holmes and Rahe 1967; Brown and Harris 1978) and can include bereavement, retirement, redundancy and so on. Life events are likely to be associated with role change. People with a broad range of social roles available to them have more flexibility to cope with a disruption to their lives than people with a more limited range of roles.

Another consequence of having a multiplicity of roles is the ability to call on more social support – to 'access' more friendship and companionship. This availability of a range of social roles and support can act as a buffer against the misfortunes and vagaries of life. We know that the availability of social support and a multiplicity of roles can help prevent people from being negatively affected by life events, and that rates of both physical and mental health problems (especially depression) are lower amongst people with higher levels of social support and a greater range of social roles to occupy. We also know that an increased frequency of stressful life events has been found in the history of people with dementia (Amster and Krauss 1974; Orrell and Bebbington 1995). It seems reasonable to suggest, then, that it is the availability of social support and the range, value and diversity of social roles available to a person that are important in determining that person's risk of developing dementia. We would suggest that education, social class and the other factors that we have highlighted act as buffer factors to lessen the effects of stress that people experience and decrease the likelihood of dementia.

There is another important factor here that relates to social role. It is through the roles that we play that we have a sense of who we are, and it is this sense of who we are – our identity – that is especially put at risk by dementia. For any one individual, the effect of this role loss – and hence the amount of intrapsychic damage – is also likely to be bound up with the degree to which the person's identity is composed of these lost roles. Thus, while role loss will be a negative factor in its own right, its effect can be magnified by the extent to which the lost roles define the person's identity.

For example, two people may lose certain skills such as knitting or driving. One may see this as a devastating loss of competence, another as a neutral facet of growing old. Where there is felt identity loss, this will lead to

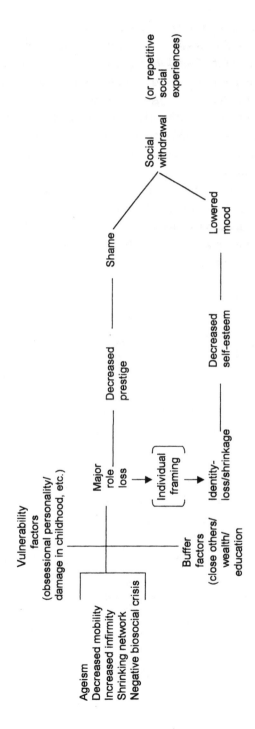

Figure 7.2 A model of the development of dementia

Source: Bender and Wainwright (1998a; 1998b)

decrease in self-esteem and depressed mood, and may well precipitate social withdrawal.

Role loss brings with it many other changes, all of which can have a cumulative effect. For instance, it disrupts established ways of time structuring and relating. Therefore, a person who has an inflexible style of coping is more likely to be at a disadvantage and at greater risk of being unable to take on new roles. An obsessional personality would be a vulnerability factor, increasing the risk of dementia. There is some empirical evidence for this. Oakley (1965) interviewed the relatives of patients on their premorbid personalities and found a greater frequency of obsessional traits compared to controls.

These factors and their relationship are visually presented in Figure 7.2. With role loss, too, comes decreased stimulation, as the person is interacting with fewer others in fewer shared activities. There is therefore decreased use of cognitive, linguistic and social skills. With decreased social interaction, there is less pressure on the person to orientate themselves toward ongoing events (*see* Figure 7.3).

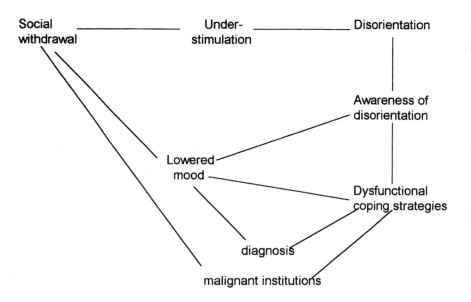

Figure 7.3 Vicious spiral of social withdrawal and disorientation
Source: Bender and Wainwright (1998a; 1998b)

With fewer interactions, the structure of their day and of their week loses coherence. One day or one week is much the same as another day or another week. Thus the distinctiveness of their time structure weakens. The person, therefore, moves into a state of decreased orientation to time and place.

As this happens, they may become alarmed at this disorientation. This may bring into play coping mechanisms such as denial, further social withdrawal to avoid embarrassment, blaming others for lost objects, etc. Whilst such coping mechanisms may succeed in decreasing the awareness of deterioration, they are not reality-grounded and therefore distort the person's perceptions and understanding of events, compounding their actual disorientation.

The person is likely to have low mood. This also reinforces social withdrawal, further reducing the person's level of stimulation. A potent vicious spiral is now in play.

Clinical Examples

Mr G was a bank manager of many years standing, of a cautious, obsessional nature. The bank was taken over and the new organisation's managers demanded higher achievements and targets, and a more ruthless style of management than Mr G felt desirable or could deliver. He went sick with stress, at which point he was offered early retirement, which he unwillingly took. Within two years he experienced memory difficulties.

Mrs K was a lady of few interests, but much enjoyed her shop assistant role. Soon after retirement she needed a cataract operation, which failed and made her eyesight worse. This prevented her from undertaking her two major – indeed only – interests of knitting and reading. Soon afterwards, her 'short-term' memory for telephone calls became very poor and conversation became repetitive.

Mr Z had a very similar set of difficulties that arose when he (eventually) retired from farming at the age of 70. He felt without a purpose and became quite depressed. A visit to a psychiatrist to discuss his inability to put names to faces or to follow conversations produced a diagnosis of dementia.

Depression, role loss and dementia

One source of evidence that supports our belief that the availability of social roles helps determine a psychosocial risk of developing dementia comes from the finding of an association between depression and dementia. This is important because the availability of a wide range of social roles is well established as a buffer against the effects of life events leading to depression.

Depression is, indeed, common amongst people with dementia. Allen and Burns, in their very thorough review paper: 'The non-cognitive features of dementia' (1995), give a figure of 30.4 per cent for symptoms of depression and 19 per cent for depressive syndrome (the equivalent figures for community controls are 8.15 per cent and 1 per cent).

Moreover, there is some suggestion that depression may act as a risk factor for dementia, which again supports our suggestion that it is the intervening variable of loss of social roles that is important. Agbayewa (1986) compared 188 patients with Alzheimer's disease and 80 patients without dementia and found that the Alzheimer's disease patients were significantly more likely to have had a psychiatric illness such as unipolar depression and paranoid disorders *earlier* in their lives. Similarly Kral (1983) and Reding, Haycox and Blass (1985) both report that when older people who have been diagnosed as having a depressive illness were followed up after a number of years, a higher level of dementia was found than would otherwise have been expected.

Dementia and cross-cultural studies

If we look at cross-cultural data, then we can find further support for this position. Richards (1997) recently reviewed the available cross-cultural studies, including those showing a very low rate of dementia in some countries in the developing world such as Nigeria (Osuntoken *et al.* 1992; Hendrie *et al.* 1995), where there is a far greater level of communal living.

In those countries or cultures making a transition towards potentially more stressful and less well-supported communities, higher rates have been found. Ineichen (1997), has attributed the increase of dementia in China, shown in more recent studies, to the move towards capitalism. Similarly, Pollitt (1997) has discussed the high rate of dementia among aboriginal Australians, who have been subject to the stresses arising from racial discrimination.

Gurland *et al.* (1983), in a careful comparison of samples in New York and London, found:

> the relative rates for depression are much the same in the two cities while the relative rates for dementia are more than twice as high in New York as in London. (p.52)

and:

> All in all, there is no obvious explanation in these data for the excess
> dementia in New York; but perhaps some supportive evidence that there
> are not only more cases of dementia in New York than in London but
> they are probably more severe as well. (pp.57–58)

Conclusions

We have argued in this chapter that it is important to see dementia as occurring within the context of a range of psychosocial and societal factors. The
key variable linking these different themes together, we believe, is that of
social role loss, which may have many important effects on people. This is
because social roles act as a buffer against the effects of life events, and it is at
least partly, if not largely, through our social roles that we as human beings
define ourselves.

We are not trying to say that a psychological model explains all cases of
dementia. However, what we hope we have shown convincingly is that it is
quite feasible and credible that psychological factors could either explain
most or much of the variance and causation in a certain number of cases. As
Tom Kitwood has argued, social, psychological and organic factors interact
in a dialectical fashion so that dementia cannot be fully understood as an
organic illness any more than it could be as simply a social or a psychological
problem.

Summary of main points

- If we want to make sense of dementia and the thoughts and
  behaviour of a person with dementia we cannot possibly do so in
  isolation from the person's history and from society and its treatment
  of them.
- A range of psychological and social factors have been suggested as
  possible risk factors for dementia. These include a person's age and
  gender; their occupational and educational history; and their social
  class. It is important to find meaningful social and psychological
  frameworks through which to account for the effect of these factors.
- A common theme running through each of these risk factors is that
  of social roles – a factor which has been implicated in the
  development of many other physical and mental health problems.

- There are at least three ways in which social roles may have an influence on the risk of developing dementia. First, the wider the range of social roles, the more alternative means there are of maintaining self-esteem. Second, the wider the range of roles, the larger the person's social network is likely to be. Effective social support can act as a buffer against the stressful effects of life events. Finally, it is through our social roles that we gain a sense of who we are – our social identity. Therefore with role loss comes identity shrinkage.

- If social roles shrink too far then the person is likely to withdraw from the social world and their engagement with it become so limited that they are at risk of becoming disorientated.

- This model is interactive with organic changes. Neither social nor organic changes occur in isolation from each other.

CHAPTER 8

A Model of the Mind in Dementia and of Levels of Severity

If we are going to reach an understanding of what happens in dementia, then we need to have a model of the mind that, while valid for all human beings, has particular relevance to the condition known as 'dementia' and the changes clinicians have noted as the severity of dementia increases.

In this chapter we first outline a model of the mind that we believe has considerable power in explaining the constellation of behaviours that constitute dementia and then look at how it explains the difficulties that arise as the severity of the condition increases. We also look at another theoretical explanation of certain behaviours that occur with severe dementia, namely attachment theory.

Bender (1996) and Wainwright (1998a; 1998b) have made a first attempt at developing a model of the mind with particular reference to dementia. They use the somewhat out of favour term 'mind' because their model makes no reference to brain functions and no attempt to localise types of mental processes in the brain. As such this is quite a different model of dementia to that which is more usually put forward – it is not about separating out one category of dementia from another or defining the nature of neurological damage within the brain. This model does not attempt to describe in exact terms the form of memory loss inflicted by neurological change. Instead Bender and Wainwright's model represents an attempt to make a link between our understanding of the damage done by the disease process and the subjective experiences of dementia.

From their clinical work, they did not see memory dysfunction as the central feature of dementia. Rather, they have suggested that people diagnosed as having dementia have great difficulty thinking and responding.

They complain of damaged skills, and may, for example, have problems planning a holiday or signing a cheque. They find themselves not knowing where they are. Symonds' (1981) definition of dementia runs along similar lines:

> It is worth summarising exactly what is meant by dementia. It is a deterioration of intellect, so that the power of creative and intelligent thought is progressively diminished. (p.1708)

So what is most centrally damaged in dementia is the ability to process information. Moreover, the loss of this ability further threatens a person's capacity to engage in socially valued roles. Both information processing and psychosocial changes act to threaten a person's senses of identity and self-worth.

It is important to realise that a system that processes information incompletely does not equate with a system that is (only) working slowly. If that were the case, then when talking to a person with dementia, all we would have to do is wait a little longer for them to reply to us! Rather, it will more usually be as if half the information is missing, making it more difficult for the person with dementia to understand what is happening around them or to communicate with others. So we are trying to make sense of an under-functioning cognitive system, not just a slow one.

Part of the loss of information processing ability (or more exactly, the loss of certain aspects of that ability) almost certainly relates to a general ageing process, and is independent of dementia. Or, looked at alternatively, the losses incurred by a person with dementia are partly attributable to their ageing, their place within a social system and their personal history. We stress once again that this is an interactive process between many different factors.

The key systems: Meaning and Safety

Bender and Wainwright's model focuses on two systems: a Meaning System and a Safety System. Figure 8.1 gives a schematic representation of the systems.

The *Meaning System* is a linguistic/conceptual system that takes the low-level configurations of sensory stimuli and interprets them in terms of previously acquired information and values. This interpretation can concern the quality of one's performance in terms of personal standards or in terms of peer or sub-group standards. Thus the Meaning System can have an impact upon emotional evaluations. For instance, it mediates depression by

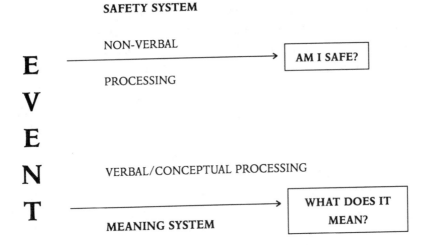

Figure 8.1 Safety and Meaning Systems
Source: Adapted from Bender and Wainwright (1998a; 1998b)

comparing present performances with previously established standards of personal competence.

The *Safety System*, in contrast, is a non-verbal perceptual system and utilises the autonomic nervous system. Its primary purpose is to maintain the physical and psychological integrity of the organism. It is sensitised to stimuli indicating danger or threat and generates a rapid choice between a small number of alternative behaviours. It is this system that is involved in initiating the fight/flight response, for instance, in which the parasympathetic nervous system is activated to increase symptoms of adrenaline in the blood supply, inhibiting the digestive system, releasing sugar into the blood so as allow energy to be made available, and so on.

Because of its rapid response and importance to survival, if activated, the Safety System's (choice of) response takes precedence over possible responses that might be generated by the Meaning System. The predominant emotions experienced by the person when the Safety System is activated are those of anxiety or fear. At certain times, however, these can also be interpreted as pleasurable events – after all, it is the same system that is involved when we watch a horror movie or take a fairground ride. In these cases it is input from the Meaning System that enables us to interpret the same bodily experiences as excitement rather than fear.

The Meaning System, then, relates to concepts, words and thought; the Safety System relates to the autonomic nervous system, the large muscles and the skeleton. It is not concerned with developing thought or action. Its sole purpose is to maintain the physical and psychological integrity of the individual. Note the use of the term 'psychological' – our Safety System is aroused not only by charging rhinos but also by an unexpected job loss or not knowing where our children are.

Whether the Safety System is activated or not is the result of the interaction between a person's felt level of resources relating to a particular situation. For example, if I am a good swimmer, a medium-size wave will not throw my Safety System; a novice, out of their depth, could well find that it activates theirs.

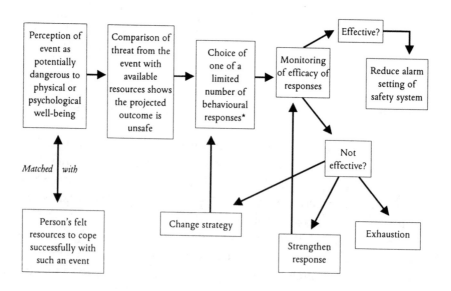

*such as flight/fight/freeze/obeisance

Figure 8.2 The Safety System
Source: Bender and Wainwright (1998c)

There is an interaction between the two systems, so that an initially frightening situation can be reinterpreted as being safe, for example when a 'stranger' approaches you on a dark walk home but on closer inspection turns out to be a friend.

Finally, note the Exhaustion variable. We think this has two purposes:

1. As a cut-out to stop the organism exhausting itself so much that it risks permanent injury or death.

2. By breaking the response sequence it gives the Meaning System the opportunity to analyse what is happening and bring its strategies to bear.

The channels of communication between the systems are two-way. The Meaning System is informed when the Safety System is activated and operating. ('Insight' may be well defined as the accuracy with which the Meaning System hypothesises what has fired the Safety System.) This ability of the Safety System to 'inform' the Meaning System becomes of considerable importance as disorientation increases.

This information processing model of what goes wrong in dementia is one way of understanding how dementia can increase in severity. As the severity of difficulties increases, so we start seeing some of the ways of handling and coping that may on the surface seem to be bizarre.

The progress of dementia: holding on

We can separate out four stages or levels of difficulty as the information processing system becomes increasingly damaged. We are aware that we have criticised the concept of stages in Chapter 4, and in recent work Bender (1998b) has re-worked the model independent of any concept of stage. However, presentation by stage provides a relatively straightforward way of representing quite complex and often subtle changes, albeit at the cost of forcing these changes into something of a conceptual straightjacket.

Table 8.1 Four levels of difficulty

1. General loss of information processing ability

2. Decreased ability to enrich meaning

3. Safety system frequently activated

4. Safety system: damage to recognition ability

Early stage

At this stage there is some loss of efficiency in information processing, and it is also likely that monitoring, especially of the world around the person, is poorer than previously. This will manifest itself in terms of poor attention. The Meaning System is unaffected in its functioning. As the person matches input from and about their behaviour with what they know about themselves they are likely to experience depression and anxiety as performances are compared to the past and found wanting. Clinically, high levels of depression have been reported by many researchers working with people with dementia (cf. Teri and Wagner 1992).

However, such emotions are not inevitable. Rather, they depend on the person's framing of their present skills. Thus, if the person explains a memory lapse in terms of 'all people's memories get worse as they age', then they may have little sense of loss.

However, the ability to empathise, to take the role of the other and to understand their viewpoint may well be damaged. This is because empathy is a very complex task and requires the observation of various sources of information that might indicate the internal state of the other, and the weighting of these sources in some priority ordering (e.g. tears are more important signifiers than scratching of the ear), all of which require good channel capacity and rapid processing.

Second stage

Due to the increasing difficulty in accessing the experiential and knowledge stores of the Meaning System, the person's language and thought becomes gradually impoverished, in terms of both level of abstraction and richness of meaning. This loss of functioning in the Meaning System has two effects on the Safety System.

First, the Meaning System, as we have seen, aids in the monitoring of responses to threats. Therefore if it is damaged, the Safety System, once triggered, will be harder to deactivate. Second, the damage to the Meaning System itself may well trigger the Safety System, since such damage implies a major loss of security.

The frequent setting-off of the Safety System has important implications for morbidity and mortality. The activity of the Safety System will cause the person to go into overactivity and the stress state described by Selye (1956; 1980) as general adaptation syndrome. Such an over-aroused state continuing over a long period of time is likely to have deleterious effects on the physical well-being of the person, as well as damaging their cognitive abilities.

One response, or class of responses, may be the appearance of coping strategies such as denial, blaming others for losses or minimising the severity of difficulties. These responses may be seen as attempts at re-framing the problem to decrease its seriousness. Although they may succeed in this aim to some extent, the cost is that incoming information is distorted to fit in with these attempts and the person's perception of reality is gradually distorted. In this stage, then, we will see fewer signs of depression and more of anxiety and insecurity.

One consequence of the use of such coping strategies may be bizarre explanations of events, such as burglars being responsible for a lost handbag. this sort of explanation can be seen as a last ditch attempt by the Meaning System to give some coherence to events.

One example of this process has been provided by the Reverend Robert Davis, whose remarkable book My Journey into Alzheimer's Disease (1989) makes compelling reading for anyone trying to make sense of dementia. The degree of insight offered may well be due to the fact that the book was co-written with his wife. Here he talks of his acute anxiety, which he refers to as 'paranoia':

> Gradually, because of not hearing, not remembering, or not comp-rehending, fear swept over me as I lost more control of my circumstances. I was gripped by paranoia. The saddest part is that I became distrustful of those who loved me and had my best interest at heart.
>
> I saw what was happening in me and I could name it at the time as paranoia. However, even though I saw it happening to me, I could do nothing to stop the feelings. I worried particularly about money. There was no reason to worry about money. The church took care of me wonderfully well as they made sure that my salary continued until our very adequate disability plan took effect. I cannot imagine the pain that it caused my friends, but I know that during this time I kept asking silly questions like 'Is the insurance paid?' or other questions of this nature. I had such a great fear. I doubted my financial security. It was irrational, but I could do nothing to control the fear. After several months of constant reassurance from my friends and my wife, I am better able to deal with these paranoid feelings. If I start down the worry path about who or what is out to get me, my wife or daughter brings me back with a gentle reminder that, 'Your paranoia is talking again.'

Having experienced these feelings makes me wonder if this is the reason why people with dementia are found hoarding strange items. The loss of self, which I was experiencing, the helplessness to control this insidious thief who was little by little taking away my most valued possession, my mind, had made me especially wary of the rest of my possessions in an unreasonable way.

This paranoia that accompanies Alzheimer's makes me fearful of so many things and has completely changed my personality. Right now, I am able to recognize many of these things, but later on as the disease progresses I realize that it is going to be a burden to everyone. My goal now is to try to programme myself to let Betty worry about the things that I cannot be reasonable about. I must make more conscious effort to trust God for the future. Each time I dignify the paranoia with an action based on the improper feeling, I strengthen the hold that the paranoia has on me. Each time I face a paranoid fear and say, 'I reject you and your hold on me for my trust is in the Lord and I will not fear what men can do to me,' I have won the battle for my mind one more day. (pp.102–103)

The maintenance of social skills and social behaviour long after severe cognitive damage has occurred has been widely commented on. Thus Church and Watters report how:

One of the authors has observed two elderly women (both scoring less than three on the CAPE Information/Orientation scale) holding a 'perfect' unprompted conversation including turn taking, hand touch, eye contact, attentiveness and laughter, for 20 minutes. One was speaking dysphasic Latvian (her language of origin), the other fluently dysphasic English. (1988, p.166)

Setting aside the obvious point that comforting has a large non-verbal component, such interactions can be accounted for by the fact that while a non-verbal social language is maintained, the conversational skills which require the involvement of the Meaning System are more frequently impaired.

Third stage

By this point clear damage to the Meaning System is occurring and consequently the Safety System is now very important in determining the person's behaviour, with attempts to reduce anxiety – wandering, repeated questioning, aggression to achieve the desired results, etc. – very evident. These responses are 'primitive' because the organism cannot draw on past experiences and knowledge to initiate more mature coping strategies.

Now it is information from the Safety System that forms the bulk of the traffic between the two systems. Faced with strong signals of distress that are not being resolved, the person clings to explanations that offer any reassurance, however incredible they may be to the observer. The increased danger to self may activate memories of fear experiences from earlier days, and the present threatening experiences may be interpreted in terms of previous threats (e.g. being physically or sexually abused).

Final stage

The key event in this final stage is damage to the recognition functions of the Safety System. It is important not to confuse this kind of damage with damage to the actual perceptual systems themselves, which might cause sensory difficulties, although this may also be present. The person is now, of course, at risk, and is highly dependent on those around him or her to monitor and maintain his or her safety.

Overview

The early stages of dementia are characterised by damage to the person's information processing ability, but the two systems are still intact; in the middle period the Meaning System suffers damage; and in the late period the Meaning System barely functions. This period is characterised by increased insecurity due to severe diminution of the skills with which the person controls his or her environment. Therefore, there is a high level of activity in the Safety System, while the damaged Meaning System is powerless to prevent the triggering of the Safety System or switch it off. Such frequent activity in the Safety System is highly stressful to the organism, and may cause physical ill-effects and hasten death. Table 8.2 summarises the situation.

Table 8.2 Four levels of difficulty: implications	
1. Loss of information processing ability	• Multiple causes; no differential diagnosis possible • High levels of depression in many people experiencing this condition
2. Meaning loss	• Uncertainty about self as executive • Loss of social self ('he's a different person') reported by relatives
3. Frequent triggering of Safety System	• High levels of anxiety, inattention and restlessness
4. Loss of recognition subsystem of Safety System	• Bizarre explanations • High dependency • Low anxiety

So far we have looked at what happens as dementia becomes more severe in information processing terms. We will now turn our attention to the theory of attachment and briefly describe how it has been used to explain some of the behaviours of people with dementia. In many ways the ideas that we will be describing are very different from the ones that we have presented so far – attachment theory has its origins in psychoanalytic psychotherapy and research, not in the hard-nosed information processing that we have outlined here. But the key issue – that dementia represents a profound sense of insecurity – is the same. Attachment theory starts from this point and then goes on to sketch in some of the ways that people can react to this insecurity.

Attachment

'Attachment' refers to a set of concepts initially set out by psychoanalysts such as Bowlby (e.g. 1972) and extended by developmental psychologists including Ainsworth (e.g. Ainsworth *et al.* 1978). It was initially proposed as a way of explaining the behaviour of very young children and toddlers and their relationships with their parents (for an overview *see* Mace and Margison 1997).

Early on in their lives, infants are said to form an attachment to one or more figures. Once attachment has been established (generally to the parents and usually to the mother) the infant tends to cry when they are separated and show pleasure when their attachment figure returns; moreover, at times of stress, for instance in a strange situation, the infant will seek out their attachment figure and gain emotional reassurance from their presence. The child's efforts to search for and cling on to their attachment figures are often described as 'attachment behaviours'.

There is an extensive body of evidence to suggest that attachment security remains a key feature of relationships throughout the whole of life. In adulthood attachment relationships are critical to both continuing security and the maintenance of emotional stability (Weiss 1991). When such attachment relationships are disrupted permanently through either bereavement or separation then this can constitute a major stressor.

Attachment and dementia

Probably the most influential proponent of attachment theory as a means of understanding the emotional world of people with dementia has been Bère Miesen, a Dutch psychiatrist. Miesen (1992; 1993) has argued that the process of dementia often strips the sufferer of the ability to recognise what should be the most familiar of people and places. Consequently, the cognitive deterioration that dementia causes means that the person with dementia will, at some stage in their illness, begin to react to the world around them as if it were a new, foreign, unrecognised world, peopled by strange, unfamiliar beings. This is not just the case when the person with dementia has to live in a hospital or nursing home, but also occurs if they live at home amongst people that they have known throughout their life.

Miesen argues that this experience of being in an insecure, frightening and strange world activates similar patterns of behaviour to the attachment behaviours seen in very young children when they encounter a new situation. The child will typically look to his or her parents for reassurance. If the parents are not present then the child may cry out and search desperately for a familiar face – behaviour which is described as attachment behaviour. Not all children react in the same way, of course; some appear to become much more frightened than others. However, some degree of anxiety is understandable. Indeed, a completely incautious child who pays no attention to whether his or her parents are present may well have difficulty establishing any form of meaningful relationship in later life.

Miesen argues that just as children will look to their parents for reassurance when confronted by a strange situation, the person with dementia will look for reassurance from those around them. Moreover, as cognitive functioning is lost, more attachment behaviours may occur. At first the person may express this need for security through non-verbal behaviour such as 'shadowing' their carer, wandering or searching for a 'missing' attachment object such as their (long dead) parent. As the bond with the outside world is disrupted further by lowered levels of cognitive functioning, and as the sense of loss, unease and fear heightens, so the person with dementia will search for some other way of holding on to a sense of emotional security. Miesen describes the development of delusions about parents, and the crying, touching and searching that are such common clinical entities of dementia, as 'parent fixation' – a means of holding on to the most fundamental attachment in a person's existence.

Many people with dementia have to face the disruption of their attachment relationships because the decline in their cognitive abilities makes it harder for them to recall from memory and therefore to psychologically 'hold on' to their attachment figure when they are not physically present. Moreover, the frequent provision of respite and other services which separate the sufferer from their main carer may also disrupt these attachment relationships.

It is worth looking in some detail at Miesen's actual research. He studied 40 patients with symptoms comparable with dementia of the Alzheimer's type, aged from 64 to 90. Using a procedure adapted from developmental psychology known as the 'strange situations test', he studied the reactions of the people with dementia when they entered a strange room with their carer, and when their carer left. He also looked at the behaviour of people with dementia on the ward and measured their levels of cognitive impairment.

Miesen found that the form of attachment behaviour varied with levels of cognitive functioning (although there were important individual differences). Those individuals with higher levels of cognitive functioning cried and called after their family member when he or she left. In contrast, people with low levels of cognitive functioning tended to express their attachment through touching; this behaviour did not change when the family member announced that he or she was leaving. Those people who were more severely affected by their illness were also more likely to act as if they believed that their parents were still alive and wander through the nursing home, calling out and looking for them.

Miesen concluded that for these people with low levels of functioning the 'strange situation' of Alzheimer's disease remained constantly present, and the feeling of being unsafe had become permanent (Miesen 1993). There were thus high levels of parent fixation. For Miesen, in Alzheimer's disease the borderline between the inner world of the imagination and the outer world of reality slowly fades. Parent fixation, he argued, served the same function for people with low levels of functioning as touching their family member did for people who were less severely affected. They were both forms of attachment behaviour – behaviours in which people with dementia engaged in order to help them feel more secure and to make the experience of dementia less frightening.

People with dementia may also show strong attachments to soft toys or particular pieces of clothing in much the same way that young children have favourite teddy bears or comfort blankets. These are called 'transitional objects' because they have some of the qualities of the attachment figure and can ease the child (or in this case the person with dementia) through a separation. Podoll et al. (1992) report two case studies of patients with dementia (one with Alzheimer's disease and the other with multi-infarct dementia). Both of these patients were said to show attachment to a soft toy, and these attachments were said to fulfil the criteria of a transitional object as described by Winnicott (1976). (These criteria include: that the person assumes rights over the object; that it is affectionately cuddled; and that it must seem to the person to give warmth, to move, to have texture, or to do something that shows that it has vitality or reality of its own.)

To conclude, Miesen argues that people with dementia perceive the world as being unsafe, frightening and strange. This activates patterns of behaviour similar to the attachment behaviours seen amongst children. In the same way that children look to their parents for reassurance, so Miesen argues, the person with dementia looks for reassurance from those around him/her.

The consequences of not meeting attachment needs: the effect on physical health

We know that if a young child's needs for attachment are not met – for instance if their parents leave them for a prolonged period of time in a strange, emotionally cold environment – there can be devastating consequences. The child may refuse to eat, withdraw into themselves or show other signs of extreme distress. When this abandonment is taken to an extreme then the psychological trauma that results may impact upon the child's physical well-being to such an extent that the child becomes mute and seems to lose the will to live. On a clinical basis, such behaviour amongst people with dementia is not uncommon, especially when they are moved away from a familiar environment. Research evidence is also beginning to emerge for this process.

Wright (1994) studied the relationship between people with Alzheimer's disease and their spouses. Thirty couples were studied over two years, with outcome assessed in terms of continued in-home care, nursing home placement or the death of the Alzheimer's disease spouse. Attachment behaviour between the Alzheimer's disease victim and their spouse continues, Wright *et al.* (1995) suggest, even in the final stages of Alzheimer's disease. Spouses are sensitive to non-verbal cues and can accurately interpret subtle changes and signals, for instance the needs to be taken to the toilet or to drink, in much the same way that mothers are sensitive to the needs of their infant children. By continuing to speak to their now mute and dying partners, to stroke their hair and to comfort them, these spouses are meeting their partners' most basic psychological needs.

However, where the spouse had not been able to continue to care for the Alzheimer's disease victim who had been placed in a nursing home there was a much higher rate of death. At the end of the study, eight of the thirty spouses with dementia had died. Wright (1994) argued that whether or not the Alzheimer's disease victims died, were placed in a nursing home or remained at home could be predicted by the amount and intensity of the spouse–patient interaction, care-giver commitment and health when the study began, and the length of time since the Alzheimer's disease had been diagnosed. Thus, where there were highly positive relationships between the person with Alzheimer's disease and their spouse the Alzheimer's disease sufferers remained at home, on average, two years longer. Conversely, low levels of interaction and low care-giver commitment were associated with the death of the Alzheimer's disease sufferer over the two year period. Interpreting the results in terms of Bowlby's attachment theory, Wright speculated that those Alzheimer's disease sufferers who subsequently died may have perceived a lack of interaction as abandonment and that this, in turn, may have led to affective withdrawal which might have weakened the patients' levels of immune functioning. Wright concludes:

> If as Bowlby argues, attachment remains important throughout life and especially in crisis situations, then it seems highly probable that it is crucial for survival of cognitively impaired persons. Interactions with a familiar individual would represent the continuation of attachment. If interactions cease, afflicted spouses may sense abandonment and die just like the infants in Spitz' studies. (p.1044)

Further evidence that there is a link between the environment in which someone with dementia is cared for and their level of immune functioning is provided by Robinson (1995), who reports how a 93-year-old woman was mechanically restrained against her will. The woman died shortly afterwards, apparently from a breakdown in her immune functioning arising from this forcible restraint.

Summary of main points

- Dementia can be considered as, in part, involving damage to the information processing system of the sufferer. We have distinguished between a Meaning System and a Safety System.

- The early stages of dementia are characterised by damage to the person's information processing ability, but the two systems are still intact. Later the Meaning System suffers damage until it reaches the point where it is barely functioning. This results in increased insecurity due to the person having severely diminished skills with which to make sense of their environment. Therefore, there is a high level of activity in the Safety System, while the damaged Meaning System is powerless to prevent the triggering of the Safety System or its switching off. Such frequent activity in the Safety System is highly stressful to the organism and may cause physical ill-effects.

- Attachment theory has been widely used to understand the behaviour of young children when they are left alone by their parents. Consistent with our position, Miesen has used attachment theory to argue that dementia is essentially a strange and frightening situation that activates very deep fears and consequently a range of behaviours aimed at making the world less frightening, including what he has termed 'parent fixation'.

- If the attachment needs of young babies are not met, then this can result in a failure to thrive and, in extreme cases, even death. If the attachment needs of people with dementia are not met, then there is evidence that this too can have severe consequences.

CHAPTER 9

The Emotional World
of Dementia Sufferers

> Until you open your eyes to your own predicament you cannot see the
> extent of it. However, if opening your eyes means seeing … devastating
> limitations is it bearable? (Sinason 1992)

In our description of the information processing deficits involved in
dementia, we distinguished between damage to the two sub-systems: the
Meaning System and the Safety System. We also detailed the way in which
attachment theory has been used as a model to account for some of the
behaviour of people with dementia in terms of a reaction to a profound
underlying insecurity.

In the remaining two chapters of Part Two we will take this process a step
further – first of all, by setting out in this chapter some of the emotional
reactions of people with dementia to the neurological and social changes
involved in this illness. Such feelings include anxiety, depression and, most
especially, loss. In the second half of the chapter we will elaborate on a point
from Chapter 8, that many of the things that people with dementia say or do
– such as denial, confusion, even hallucination – can be seen as attempts to
deal with the emotional consequences of the illness and as a way of holding
on to who they are. This is the form of understanding people with dementia
need and it is to this issue that we will devote the final two parts of this book.

It is worthwhile to take a moment before we embark on this task to
outline some of the essential elements of the model that we will be putting
forward. Our argument can be simply stated:

1. The most appropriate starting point for any psychological consideration of people with dementia and the services that they need should be the subjective experience of people with dementia. This is characterised by both the experience of loss (of social roles and relationships as well as of neurological functioning) and the threat of further losses to come, and results in a range of emotions including grief, depression, anxiety, despair and terror.

2. There is some evidence that individuals who have experienced a significant loss of role or status are at greater risk of developing dementia, a process that in itself reduces the range of roles available to the individual. The experience of dementia therefore represents a profound threat to the individual's identity – to their sense of who they are.

3. People with dementia need to be seen as active agents. They are engaged in both an active struggle to cope with the threat to their identity posed by the direct and indirect effects of dementia, and an attempt to resolve or work through the emotional challenges posed by this illness.

4. The adaptive responses of people with dementia – the ways in which they attempt to cope with dementia – are often misinterpreted as further evidence of impairment. Consequently, these behavioural strategies and emotional reactions are often seen not as the responses of people to a ghastly predicament but as proof of a degenerative process occurring within the brain.

5. The social context within which people who suffer from dementia are cared for needs to be one that encourages people with dementia to cope and to manage their illness in as useful a way as they possibly can. In particular, people with dementia need to be seen as capable of both emotional growth and change, and also of maintaining a coherent identity into the later stages of the illness.

6. Services for people with dementia and their carers therefore need to be organised so that they assist in this process. They need to enable the individual to hold on to their sense of self and also to recognise the deep emotional trauma that is involved. Good patterns of dementia care will allow people with dementia to work their way through or emotionally process their experiences. For many this will take the form of grieving for their losses.

Losing oneself in dementia

In many ways people with dementia are caught in a dilemma – they have a need to make sense of their lives, but to do so is to risk being confronted by the awfulness of their situation. The starting place for any clinician, then, is to understand this dilemma – to understand the subjective experience of people with dementia.

As clinicians and as carers our key task is to understand their world through their eyes. If we can do this then we can begin to have some understanding of their understandings (however partial or confused), feelings (however incompletely or oddly expressed) and beliefs. We will begin to walk a long mile in their shoes.

We talk of feelings being 'incompletely or oddly expressed' because we recognise the possibility that the emotions of a person with dementia are not expressed as fully as those of people with intact cognitive abilities. This is what is sometimes called 'snatches of lucidity' (Balfour 1995), although 'fragmented expression' is probably a better way of framing it. To use Murray Parkes' (1975) useful phrase, our 'assumptive worlds' may be very different from theirs, and these differences may concern feelings, behaviours and/or beliefs, and their interactions.

With the cognitively able, the clinician is flooded by cues and non-verbal behaviours, and need only pick a few cues to understand where the client 'is at'. The clinician working with a person who has dementia (a) has to work with far fewer cues, and (b) even if they correctly understand the emotion, cannot 'run off' the consequent behaviours or beliefs.

For example, if your partner said that they would pick you up to go out at 7 o'clock, and by 7.20 they have not shown up, then you may be getting a bit anxious and irritated (feelings), wonder if their car has broken down (belief) and think about ringing them (behaviour). Now most people could empathise easily with these feelings and understand these behaviours and beliefs.

In contrast, the person with dementia might be completely overwhelmed with anxiety about their partner's non-appearance, create a much more unrealistic set of beliefs to account for it and behave in a way that others would find unreasonable. Moreover, while in some cases very catastrophic reactions can be precipitated by even quite trivial absences such as going to the lavatory, for other people with dementia even bereavements do not appear to be registered. So, the feelings, beliefs and behaviours of people with dementia appear to be much less predictable than those of the cognitively-intact, and relating to this unpredictability is a far more skilled job. This, of course, has implications both for the selection of staff with suitable attitudes and for their training. We will discuss this issue in Part Four.

What feelings might someone with dementia have as a result of the process that they are going through? And how might these feelings be expressed? We think it very likely that the process of having dementia will set off extremely strong emotional reactions, amongst which will often be anxiety, depression, grief and terror. Table 9.1 is an attempt to describe some of the feelings that a person with dementia might have and suggest how these feelings can be conveyed to others. The right-hand 'statements' are not totally satisfactory as they are rather stereotyped. Moreover, of course, each person will have their own unique feelings, while the strength of those feelings will vary across time, as will their ability to express those feelings.

Table 9.1 Major emotions and possible feeling statements of people who believe they have dementia	
Anxiety/fear about their future	What will happen to me? Will my spouse stay with me? Or will she/he have me put away? Will I end up in a dementia ward? Will I end up incontinent?
Grief/loss	I'm not sure I'm safe to drive I can't understand TV programmes I'm making lots of spelling mistakes I'm losing myself Friends don't call any more I can't talk to my children about what's on my mind
Depression/loss of self-esteem	I've got no energy I'm useless I'm not any good for anything I don't know why he/she puts up with me I want to die
Terror	I'll end up like them This place is a living hell I never thought I/it would end like this I'm terrified/very scared These people are very dangerous

Source: Adapted from Bender and Cheston (1997)

What we have outlined here is a descriptive frame in which we draw especial attention to the fact that extremes of emotion are likely and indeed common. We do not wish to suggest that this is an exhaustive list of the feelings engendered by the dementing process, nor that these are the only ways to conceive of the phenomena that we will describe. What we do wish to emphasise is the need to develop detailed accounts of the ways in which individuals with dementia experience this process and respond to these experiences. This is our attempt to do so, but we understand that other representations of this process are of course also possible.

Emotional responses to dementia

Grief at the loss of abilities and valued skills

> It now appears that even demented persons experience and feel threatening losses, and it would appear that the process of dementia creates an environment which fosters uncertainty and the lack of safety. This could mean that demented persons are struggling with emotional problems, which have been hitherto underestimated. (Miesen 1992, p.223)

Having dementia involves a process of losing so many things. The ability to learn and remember information, to make sense out of the world around one, to plan and carry out the decisions that one has made – all these abilities, as well as many others, decline, making day-to-day tasks harder and harder. In the majority of cases, having dementia also involves other losses and other changes in one's relationships with other people such as attending a Day Centre, the loss of self-esteem and so on.

But unlike some amnesias brought about by head injuries, for instance, these losses occur over a long period of time. For people with dementia, the awareness that they are not performing at the level that they have expected of themselves is compounded by the threat that their abilities will continue to decline over the coming months and years. Thus for people with dementia, the need to grieve for those losses that have already occurred is compounded by the threat of further losses to come.

Probably the best known theory of how people cope with loss concerns how death and dying affects people. Two influential theories have been proposed.

The first, by Colin Murray Parkes (1986), outlines a series of five stages that people who have been bereaved progress through: from shock to despair, and from there to guilt, anger and resolution. In a similar way,

Elizabeth Kübler-Ross (1970) has theorised that those who are terminally ill move from denial to anger, depression and bargaining before finally accepting the inevitability of their death.

The stage approach to grief and loss has been criticised for being too inflexible and mechanistic (Worden 1991). One of the main drawbacks of stage theories of change in general is that they can be understood to mean that any individual, at any one time, can be seen as being at one stage rather than another, and that all individuals progress smoothly from one stage to the next. As a consequence these kinds of description tend to be seen as somewhat arbitrary and rigid, and deflect attention away from the human processes that underlie them.

Nevertheless, these stage theories have the merit of making intuitive sense of much of the material, and have been very influential. It is therefore not surprising that many of the analyses of the ways in which people with dementia cope with the changes that are involved in this illness have described a series of stages (e.g. Cohen, Kennedy and Eisdorfer 1984; Keady 1997; Keady and Nolan 1994; 1995a).

For example, Cohen *et al.* (1984) describe people with dementia as moving through a series of stages. Progression through these psychological changes depends upon a number of factors, including the personality of the individual and the social world surrounding the individual. The six stages that Cohen *et al.* have set out are as follows:

Pre-diagnosis: recognition and concern

Reaction to the diagnosis: denial

anger, guilt and sadness

coping

maturation

separation from the self

The way in which people with dementia can be helped to move through this process is a point to which we will return in Part Three, when we discuss counselling and psychotherapeutic approaches to working with people with dementia.

Cohen *et al.*'s model is one of a number of descriptions of grieving amongst people with dementia which are largely an adaptation of traditional models of grieving. Often the emotional pain of the loss is said to be so threatening that the person with dementia has to adopt a series of unconscious defence mechanisms in order to shut out the emotional load of the loss from conscious awareness.

Keady and Nolan (1994) propose an eight-stage model to make sense of early onset dementia:

> slipping
>
> suspecting
>
> covering up
>
> revealing
>
> confirming
>
> surviving
>
> disorganisation
>
> decline and death

Some clinicians and psychotherapists have suggested that because of their cognitive deficit, people with dementia are not able to complete the process of grieving. Thus Solomon and Szwarbo (1992) have described the experience of grief of a person with dementia as a narcissistic injury suffered through the process of psychosis. The loss is a loss of part of the self (memory, intellect and other aspects of ego functioning). In the case of individuals without a dementing illness, losses are seen as triggering a process of grieving in which the person concerned moves through a number of stages: denial, disorganisation and, finally, reorganisation. However, Solomon and Szwarbo suggest that the person with Alzheimer's disease or another dementia is unable to move on to the final stage because of their limited brain functioning and get 'stuck' in the stage of disorganisation.

Solomon and Szwarbo maintain that the subjective experience of dementia is 'not all that different from a pathological grief response. Indeed a few never get beyond the stage of denial' (p.300). As they are unable to deal with conflict and stress so the individual goes down the path of least resistance leading to withdrawal and depression.

Depression

Grief and depression are clearly overlapping emotions. However, it may be useful to differentiate between them. For instance, Freud noted in *Mourning and Melancholia* (1917) that the person with loss has a very negative emotional tone which is shared with the depressed person but, in contrast to the depressed person, they do not necessarily blame themselves for that loss or think less of themselves.

At the heart of dementia, then, is loss. It is known that as humans we react to loss in many different ways but that the most common reaction is sadness. When the impact of these losses becomes clinically significant then a frequent psychiatric consequence is depression. It is not surprising, then, that depression has been the most commonly reported affective response of people with dementia.

Estimates of the proportion of people with dementia who are depressed vary widely, depending in part on the criteria used to define dementia in different studies. While Burns, Jacoby and Levy (1990c) found that none of the patients that they studied satisfied the DSM III R (revised) criteria for a major depressive disorder, depressive symptoms were reported nevertheless by almost two-thirds (63 per cent) of their sample. Patients were more likely to report depression than relatives and the reporting of depressive symptoms was related to the severity of the dementing illness.

However, other studies have found high levels of clinical depression. Teri and Reifler (1987) reported that approximately 30 per cent of patients with Alzheimer's disease met the DSM III criteria for major depressive disorder. If the definition of depression is relaxed then even higher rates can be found. For instance, Cummings and Victoroff (1990) estimated the prevalence of depression in people with Alzheimer's disease at up to 87 per cent.

As we described in an earlier chapter, clinical depression, whatever its origin, may act, in psychiatric terms, as a pseudodementia – that is to say, a condition which mimics the clinical pattern of dementia. Consequently, one of the most common clinical problems that is presented to mental health professionals and those in the social services who work with older adults concerns the elderly person who seems to be withdrawn, forgetful and tearful or in low spirits. The question that is commonly asked concerns whether this memory loss can best be thought of as being a result of clinical depression or a sign that the person has a dementing illness. The two clinical diagnoses tend to be seen as two separate entities. In many ways, separating out the apparent decline in the person's cognitive functioning caused by dementia from any changes in their emotional state arising from non-organic causes is an impossible feat: it is perfectly possible for the two to co-exist.

Indeed, as we suggested earlier in Chapter 7, there is some evidence that depression may be a risk factor for dementia; and that depression may reflect the loss of role and status. But it is probably also the case that the factors that produce depression also predispose a person to develop dementia; that cognitive and emotional decline interact in a cumulative fashion so that depression is aggravated by social and neurological changes; and that in turn, depression makes it harder for a person with dementia to withstand continued neurological deterioration.

Anxiety

For people with dementia, the threat of continued change and decline is profound. Indeed, it is perhaps no exaggeration to suggest that one of the greatest fears within Western society is that, as we age, we may not only become increasingly physically infirm but also enter a personal hell of progressive mental deterioration. For many, the slightest lapse in memory may thus become a cause for concern. Even when intellectual deterioration is such that a diagnosis of probable dementia is reached, the mental health professionals who make the diagnosis will not be able to predict the speed of decline or its severity, only that decline is inevitable.

For some people with dementia, this threat will be experienced not within a safe, reassuring world where those around that person are willing to discuss the issues involved, but within an atmosphere of silence in which the future is too unsafe to be mentioned. Dementia has become such a taboo subject that it may seem that the issue cannot be discussed. It is not unusual for those around the person to be unwilling to give him or her the diagnosis; for the spouse to be given information that is withheld from the sufferer; and for the sufferer to be given false explanations for changes in his or her lifestyle – for example being told that attending a day hospital will help them with a minor physical condition. This is part of the malignant social psychology that Kitwood has described (e.g. Kitwood 1990a; Kitwood and Bredin 1992).

It is hardly surprising, then, that people who have been given a diagnosis of dementia often become anxious, suspicious and, on occasion, even paranoid. Indeed, anxiety and its associated psychiatric variants are consequently a frequently-reported accompanying feature of dementia. Solomon and Szwarbo (1992), for instance, report that of the 86 people assessed by Solomon, 49 could be described as having a non-specific anxiety, with yet others having more specific fears and panic attacks.

Despair or terror

Dementia is not simply an illness. The erosion of mental abilities represents the potential destruction of the person. People with dementia can experience a profound, existential sense of emptiness and absence, related to the actual or anticipated damage to their sense of self. The deep despair and terror that this sense of absence can engender can be compounded by neglect by those around the person. Much of the behaviour of professionals they meet – the extended assessments, the frequent failure to offer emotional support and nurturance to the sufferers themselves – can be seen as the avoidance behaviour of people who cannot refuse to interact with people with dementia but wish to avoid contamination. This means that there are few safe places in which the person with dementia can explore this process and begin to make sense of the phenomenological reality of dementia.

The poor functional performance of people with dementia is understandable, to a considerable extent, in terms of their emotional reactions. Rather than being due to some mysterious, remorseless organic process, the person's performance is a response to their terror – a terror fuelled by their partly remembered, partly suppressed memories of the treatment of people who have dementia. The precise nature of their future may be unpredictable, but their near complete social devaluation – Goffman's (1963) term 'spoilt identity' is very apposite – is highly predictable, as is the likelihood of their being involved with poorly-financed, poorly-run services using predominantly untrained and poorly-paid staff.

We will return to this theme of dementia as posing a threat to a person's identity in the next chapter.

Coping with loss of identity

Coping with loss and the threat of loss

Human beings have to deal with loss and the threat of loss in many different forms, from bereavement to redundancy or the loss of health. The person with dementia copes with their illness within the context of a reduced cognitive capacity and often a restricted social world. But the behaviour of the person with dementia is not so different from the behaviour of other people who are also having to cope with profound change.

When we look, in this chapter, at how people with dementia cope with what is happening to them, we will continue to emphasise one of the themes established earlier in this book – that of seeing the behaviour and talk of people with dementia as meaningful. In particular, we want to explain how many of the behaviours that are seen as being typical of dementia (such as lengthy reminiscences, delusions and aggression), which are routinely attributed to the actions of the disease process on the brain, can be better understood as arising from the strategies that people with dementia use as a means of coping with what is happening to them.

With any form of coping, regardless of the exact nature of the threat that exists, a balance needs to be struck between shutting-out from awareness all sense of threat and being completely overwhelmed by it. At first people tend to respond by using coping strategies that involve shutting-off the threat or diverting their attention away from it. As the threat is established and becomes more evident, so the balance shifts and the threat is gradually incorporated into the person's view of him- or herself and the world. The alternative to using such strategies would be to live in either a world in which we could not make sense out of our lives or a world of traumatic levels of emotional distress. For most people neither course is tolerable for long.

The way in which a person with dementia copes with their experiences is likely to be influenced by a number of factors including: the pattern of their neurological deterioration; their previous psychological health; the quality of care that they receive; other losses in their lives; and their previous styles of coping.

PREVIOUS STYLES OF COPING

A significant theme within much of the therapeutic work with older adults over the last thirty years has been the belief that, as individuals age, so they face common life tasks (cf. Erikson 1977; 1985). Failure to complete these life tasks adequately has been seen as threatening the person's future psychosocial stability. Thus, in order to understand people in late life, including people with dementia, it is necessary to see them in the context of their whole life history, with crises from earlier stages in their lives both successfully and unsuccessfully resolved. On a similar theme, it is likely that where an individual has had a traumatic experience earlier in their life they are likely to interpret the trauma of dementia in these terms. Thus Miesen and Jones (1997) relate the resurfacing of psychic pain in dementia to traumas experienced earlier in life, for instance during war. They argue that the experience of alienation from others and ultimately from oneself that dementia brings is essentially similar to earlier traumas. People with dementia will try to make sense of their experiences by seeing them in terms of past traumas.

Consequently, as a general rule, those individuals who can be thought of as in some way more psychologically healthy before the onset of the illness should be able to deal with the process of neurological damage involved in dementia more adaptively than would psychologically dysfunctional individuals.

In particular, it is likely that the coping strategies that an individual uses during at least the initial stages of the illness will be those that were in habitual use before the illness. If the person with dementia has tended to try to shut out painful information then it will be harder for him or her to address present losses.

PREVIOUS LOSSES

People with dementia deal with many other losses as well as those involved in the dementing process itself, such as sensory loss, loss of home and loss of social contacts. Elsewhere in the clinical literature it has been found that psychiatric disturbance increases in proportion to the severity of multiple losses (Holmes and Rahe 1967; Murphy 1986). It is not just that the loss and its subsequent handicap creates emotional disturbance as part of its process, but also that the burden of a handicap depletes the individual's resources, leaving him or her prey to what is internally unresolved and disturbed (Sinason 1992). The effects of these losses, however, may well be mitigated, depending on the extent to which the person with dementia receives support from those around him or her.

A common means by which people handle threatening events is denial. As this is often found in clinical reports of people with dementia, we will now consider it in some detail.

Denial or a lack of insight

Denial and insight are difficult concepts, as it is almost always the person with the greater status or power in a relationship who defines what is to count as 'the reality' against which the dementia sufferer's response will be measured. For instance, David (1990) suggests that insight can be considered to have three related aspects:

- the ability to re-label various mental events as pathological
- the recognition by the patient that he or she has a mental illness
- the extent to which he or she complies with the appropriate medical treatment for that illness.

From David's description we can see that anything that falls short of a complete acceptance of the state of affairs as defined by other people could be construed as amounting to a lack of insight. For people with dementia, having complete 'insight' into their condition in David's terms would represent an enormous emotional challenge. They would have to acknowledge that their behaviour is abnormal and that they have a dementing illness, and be prepared to accede to whatever changes in their lifestyle that appear to be necessary. It is unsurprising, then, that many people with dementia refuse to view themselves in this light!

There is another problem with viewing insight in these terms. It tends to be seen as something that resides within a person – something that they have or don't have. We would argue that it may be more useful to think of insight and denial as coping mechanisms that are used within the context of the world around the person with dementia, and we will elaborate this view in the next few pages.

Thinking of denial as a psychological defence mechanism rather than simply a facet of neurological deterioration has led a number of researchers to attempt to find out whether people with dementia who are in a state of denial are less anxious or depressed than those who are not using this defence mechanism and who would be thought of as having a more 'realistic' view of their illness. There is some evidence that amongst people with dementia the use of denial is inversely related to depression (e.g. Sevush and Leve 1993) and anxiety (e.g. Verhey *et al.* 1993). Cotrell and Lein (1993) interviewed the spouses of five people with dementia, and with one exception, the more 'realistic' the dementia victim's perceptions of the problem, the more depressed he or she was said to be. The dementia sufferers' denial did not relate simply to their illness – whereas three of the five sufferers were described as using fantasy as a way of escaping the reality of their present circumstances, one was reported as having erased all memories of a previous, unhappy period in his life.

Clearly, there are enormous differences in the ways in which people with dementia are able to talk about what it is like to have dementia. Bahro et al. (1995) presented a series of seven case studies describing how drug trial participants who had diagnoses of Alzheimer's disease coped with their illness. The authors detailed how the group of patients used a variety of defence mechanisms, including partial or complete denial:

... some patients avoided naming their illness or did not seek out any information about it. In addition, other patients exhibited dissociation of affect, vagueness and circumstantiality in discussing their condition. Some minimised the severity of their functional impairment. Further mechanisms of defence included externalisation, displacement, somatisation and self-blame. Only one patient (case 7) did not exhibit any of these mechanisms. She was more aware of her illness at both a cognitive and emotional level and coped more adequately by a process of appropriate mourning. (p.45)

We believe that it is more useful to consider denial as one of a number of coping mechanisms that arise from the interaction between the person and the world around them, and consequently that denial should be considered as both functional and variable.

DENIAL IS FUNCTIONAL

We need to think of denial in terms of the functions that it serves and evaluate its use in terms of its effectiveness in meeting those functions. For many people with dementia, it is just too awful to have to think about what is happening to them. Often, denying that they have dementia is a way in which people with dementia can protect themselves against something that is simply too traumatic to be able to deal with. Denial prevents the individual being overwhelmed by the emotional consequences of the losses that they have suffered or the threat that the dementing process represents.

Denial is thus the equivalent of a psychological time-out – it can provide individuals with time in which they can develop other strategies of coping which will be more effective. Denial is not a particularly effective coping strategy, as it leaves the person isolated from reality and unable to explain many of the things that are occurring. All around them may be evidence that they cannot account for. Unfortunately it is a strategy that can become habitual. We would expect to see denial become a habitual and semi-permanent means of coping when the threat seems immense and the person seems to have few resources (either personal or social) with which to deal with them. Consequently, Tom Kitwood has described denial or a lack of insight as a possible indication of an impoverished care environment.

DENIAL IS VARIABLE

Denial, then, is a coping strategy which we would expect people to use on a long-term basis only if and when the environment around them is continually not safe enough to allow them to explore their experiences, and/or when the individual lacks the personal resources to engage more meaningfully with the world about them. Consequently, denial is a strategy which will be used some times but not at others, and concern some aspects of cognitive loss but not others – depending partly on the social context. The dementia sufferer's awareness of their losses, therefore, can be seen as a response which can potentially be influenced by people and events around the person.

We can see various levels of denial being used by people with dementia:

- *Complete denial of all problems or difficulties.* Although this insulates the individual from any awareness of the difficulties they face, it isolates the individual from a reality which will not go away and is consequently difficult to sustain in the face of continued evidence to the contrary.

- *Acknowledging a problem but attributing its cause to a benign influence* (for instance, seeing a memory problem as part of normal ageing). While more adaptive than complete denial, again this strategy can be difficult to maintain in the face of evidence to the contrary. It can also take the person with dementia into disagreement with the interpretations of powerful professionals.

- *Acknowledging a problem but denying its implications.* Here the person with dementia acknowledges that they have difficulties but does not admit their need for specialist help.

- *Emotional denial* (often referred to as 'intellectualisation'). Here the individual is able to talk about his or her difficulties, but does not allow him- or herself to become emotionally involved with the material.

Balfour (1995) found that people with Alzheimer's disease, when making up stories to account for what was happening in an ambivalent picture that they had been asked to comment upon, referred significantly more often than the control group to the theme of 'handicap'. The most consistent references to this theme were made by those people at the lower level of functioning. It is likely that many of these people would, nevertheless, in David's (1990) terms, have been thought to have lacked insight. Yet these indirect expressions of loss allow material to be emotionally processed in a relatively unthreatening manner. By talking in this way about loss, these people with dementia may have been able to express something about what it was like to have dementia and to begin to work through their feelings. This is an issue that we will deal with in more detail in our discussion of therapeutic intervention in Part Three.

Let us turn to other means of managing the environment and its terrifying messages about one's lack of well-being.

Avoidance – becoming confused

Dementia is sometimes described as a confusional state, as if being confused was an inevitable part of having dementia. But confusion is a common human experience. We all are liable to become confused when our capacity to retain and make sense of information is overloaded. For people with dementia this may occur more often – after all, their capacity to retain and to process information is reduced. But confusion is *not* inevitable. Moreover, confusion, like denial, can be considered as a coping strategy – often it is better to be confused about the world than to have its realities laid bare.

Fantasy and the imagination

Hallucinations and delusions are frequently associated with dementia. Burns *et al.* (1995) found evidence of hallucinations in 17 per cent of their 178 subjects, while reports of delusions amongst people with dementia vary from 16 per cent (Burns, Jacoby and Levy 1990a), to 37 per cent (Berrios and Brook 1985) and 50 per cent (Cummings *et al.* 1987). Auditory hallucinations are consistently reported at between 50 and 70 per cent of the frequency of visual hallucinations (Allen and Burns 1995). The appearance of psychotic symptoms such as delusions and hallucinations are often associated with a subsequent accelerated cognitive decline. Consequently, hallucinations or delusions tend to be ascribed directly to the process of neurological deterioration.

For some people with dementia, present reality is so threatening that they recall a time in life which was less disturbing and disquieting. This is one of the reasons for what is often described as temporal disorientation, in which the person with dementia seems to imagine that they are in a different time or period of their life. Related to this is the way in which some people with dementia recall to life through their imagination significant people from their past, such as their parents or their husband or wife. It is as if they are helping themselves to feel secure by re-creating a person who will rescue them from their current emotionally unstable world. 'If only', they seem to be saying, 'if only my dear Sidney was still alive, he wouldn't let me suffer in this way.' This means of coping with the threat that dementia poses involves what psychoanalysts would term projection and wish fulfilment.

Thus, if the person with dementia has to deal with the death of his or her spouse, then this loss may be experienced in terms of the loss of an original attachment figure, leading to the delusion that as well as the sufferer's husband or wife, a parent has recently died. Moreover, the fact that delusions of theft and suspicion are amongst the most commonly reported delusions may reflect the projection of an underlying sense of loss. An awareness at a conscious level of both the effects of an illness and of changes within social relationships may awake deep fears of abandonment – a 'dis-ease' with life. This anxiety may be reflected in accusations towards the spouse which appear to others as paranoia or jealousy (Cotrell and Lein 1993).

Externalising the cause of one's problems – blaming others

Part of the process, then, by which people with dementia cope with loss and the threat of loss is to attribute the causes of their difficulties to others, and in particular their spouses or carers. We described in an earlier chapter how, in response to the terror of cognitive loss, people with dementia may cling to those who are nearest to them or search for those attachment figures, perhaps even re-creating them through fantasy. Yet the relationship between carer and sufferer is a complex one: for the carer, there are many emotions and strains, including guilt, resentment and depression; for the sufferer, their dependence on another is a two-edged sword, and the emotional security that their carer may provide is, at most, only a temporary solution. *The person whose presence provides relief is the same person who may leave one on one's own.* Indeed, the very fact of being so dependent on another is a reminder of how much life has changed, of that which has been lost and of the losses that may occur in the future.

Where the person with dementia makes accusations about their spouse or carer, then, they do so within what is often a complex and shifting emotional world. Moreover, the blaming of others for one's own difficulties may well be reinforced by the relief from psychological strain that it provides. Externalising the cause of their difficulties allows people with dementia to represent these difficulties as temporary and capable of resolution.

When words are not enough – aggression as a means of expressing feelings

Blaming others often leads to verbal and at times physical violence by people with dementia against their carers. Arguably, of all the behaviours associated with dementia, this is the hardest one for carers to deal with. It is not just the pain arising from the blow – the hurt is as much emotional as it is physical. Unfortunately, aggressive behaviour is also relatively common. Burns, Jacoby and Levy (1990c) concluded that predominantly physical, as opposed to verbal, aggression occurred in around 20 per cent of people with dementia.

A number of studies have found an association between levels of aggression and cognitive decline associated with an underlying neurological deficit. For instance, Burns *et al.* (1990c) found that patients who were aggressive were significantly more cognitively impaired than those who were not aggressive. In particular, they found that aggression was associated with damage to the temporal lobes. Similarly, Volkow and Tancredi (1987) described four cases of repetitive, purposeless violent behaviour, all of whom showed evidence of abnormalities in the left temporal lobe. Attempts have also been made to link aggression with one form or another of dementia, but these remain inconclusive (Ryden 1988).

Aggressive behaviour can also be seen as reflecting the dementia sufferer's increasing frustration at being unable to communicate or to comprehend. Thus Welsh, Corrigan and Scott (1996) found a highly significant negative correlation between carers' assessments of the aggression of their partners and the ability of the person with dementia to use language to express themselves.

People with dementia may be unable to respond to the difficulties their situation presents by initiating affectionate actions which will allow their carers to behave in a similar way. Such reciprocal turn-taking would allow the attachment needs of both carer and sufferer to be met. But instead, the sufferer reacts in a catastrophic or aggressive manner, arguing with their carer or blaming them for their problem. Thus a problem which may have been resolved peaceably and without difficulty develops into a major crisis.

Aggression and other secondary symptoms such as fear, restlessness and sadness have also been represented as reactions to the psychological losses associated with dementia (Miesen 1995). As a means of defence against these losses individuals with dementia may externalise the blame for their condition. Anger directed at others will cause the patient to suspect the motives of others, and this suspiciousness can then be aggravated and entrenched by memory and sensory deficits (Solomon and Swarbo 1992).

This would account for the finding of an association between aggression and the development of delusions, as the content of the delusions may partly represent the projections of painful attachment issues (Cooper, Mungas and Weiler 1990; Flynn, Cummings and Gorbein 1991; Lachs *et al.* 1992).

Penny – an angry woman

One of the most fundamental means of gaining emotional reassurance is through sensual and physical intimacy. It is through being held and holding onto others, being touched and touching our loved ones that we can reassure ourselves of our own attractiveness, our potency and, perhaps most importantly of all, that we are loved and that we can love.

One woman, Penny, that one of us worked with, was referred because she was frequently angry with her husband, attacking him both verbally and physically. When she attacked him, she would often accuse him of having secret affairs (all of which her husband tearfully denied) and would demand to know the names of his lovers. In some sense Penny only seemed to be continuing with a pattern that she had established earlier in her life, before she began to suffer from dementia, in which she was always very jealous of her husband's behaviour.

Like many people with dementia, Penny seemed to have a great need for emotional comfort and reassurance and she relied on her husband to supply this. At times these needs took the form of requests and demands for sexual intercourse, and her husband told the Community Psychiatric Nurse that Penny was far more keen to make love than he was. After they had made love, Penny was much more tender and compassionate towards him than at other times. Normally she followed him around the house and would hardly let him out of her sight, angrily attacking him if he left her, even to visit the toilet. However, after they had made love, she would allow him to wander around the house as he wanted without attempting to follow him.

Wright *et al.* (1995) cite Hall and Buckwalter (1987) as ascribing rage that is out of proportion to a simple request or incident to a 'Progressively Lowered Stress Threshold' (PLST). They suggest that situations which may appear normal to cognitively intact persons can be confusing and highly uncontrollable for cognitively impaired persons. Hall and Buckwalter suggest that by reducing confusing environmental stimuli, stress and anxiety can be reduced and catastrophic reactions diminished.

Aggressive behaviour needs to be understood as potentially serving a function within a social context. It is a form of communication, albeit an exceptionally difficult one for carers to deal with.

The social context of emotional behaviour

Emotions are not simply internal, personal and subjective feelings. They can also be understood as actions in a social world. The relationship between emotional behaviour and the social environment is reciprocal: emotional behaviour occurs within a social context, but emotions also provide the context through which actions and language can be understood. For instance, there is a world of difference between a friendly slap on the back between colleagues and an angry push in a bus queue, even though the behaviour itself may be very similar. Thus, if we do not understand the emotional world of people with dementia, then we will be unable to understand fully their social behaviour: it will appear to be meaningless or we will be liable to mis-understand it.

This is the reason, then, why so many of the reactions and coping strategies of people with dementia that we have described in the last two chapters are so frequently misinterpreted. Instead of being seen as displays of emotional behaviour they are wrongly attributed to neurological damage and cognitive deficit. The observer simply does not look at this behaviour through an empathic perspective.

We can think of emotional behaviour as a continuum. At one end of the continuum people are able to reflect upon and think through their experiences. At the other end of the continuum emotional behaviour is not a matter of reflecting upon such experiences, and is instead expressed physically and immediately. An example of this second type is where a person with dementia cries out for their (dead) mother, the behaviour that Miesen has described as parent fixation.

People with dementia, then, can be thought of as moving from being able to reflect upon and re-create their experiences towards the immediate display of emotions. In part, this movement is due to the process of cognitive decline. Additionally, and more importantly in the context of dementia care, the degree to which this transition occurs is a function of the social environment in which these emotional displays take place.

The extent to which people can show their emotions is regulated by the social system in which they are located. In systems where there is strong social control the display of strong emotions is discouraged. Such displays tend to be seen as being in 'bad taste' and people feel uncomfortable with them; emotional behaviour is thus limited. Conditions that are receptive to the expression of strong emotional behaviours have been obtained in special therapeutic circumstances (such as encounter groups or drama therapy), but can be experienced as threatening or uncontained by people who are unused to such strong emotional behaviour.

Good dementia care involves being open to all forms of emotional actions. It involves, in essence, the holding and containment of the emotional content of an action and its reflection back in a form that can be used by the patient. We need to be open to both the emotional content of reminiscences and the despairing need for reassurance shown in parent fixation and other attachment behaviours, and even in aggression. We will address these issues in more depth in Chapter 13.

To date the most comprehensive attempt to define dementia care from a psychological perspective has been Dementia Care Mapping. This defines good dementia care in terms of care practices that respect and value an individual's 'personhood', and thus sees good care as essentially therapeutic. We would argue that there is a need to take this process of care one step further and address the issue of psychotherapeutic change with people with dementia. In the next part of this book we will turn our attention to the way in which care for people with dementia should be organised.

Summary of main points

- The starting point for any psychological understanding of dementia has to be the experiences of people who suffer from this illness.
- People with dementia experience both the loss of a range of abilities and roles and the threat of future negative changes.
- People with dementia experience a range of strong emotions including anxiety, terror, grief and depression.
- These emotions are not static. They change and it is possible for people with dementia to work through them.
- The methods of coping that we have outlined in this chapter can be thought of as avoidance or deflection strategies. Through their use the threat that dementia represents can be pushed away, avoided or deflected, with the result that the person's view of themselves alters little to take account of their new position.

- Although these strategies can be effective, if the person with dementia persists with them over an extended period of time then their ability to interact effectively in the world will be greatly reduced. It is a bit like burying one's head in the sand – the problem itself does not go away.

- It is often thought that people with dementia use denial as a means of dealing with loss, and that they consequently lack insight. However, denial, like all coping strategies, needs to be seen as both functional and variable.

- Other deflection strategies include avoidance, fantasy and blaming others.

- The social context within which many people with dementia live is dominated by the organic model of dementia. This emphasises organic determinants of behaviour and does not see people with dementia as emotional beings. As a consequence the behaviour of people with dementia is often misinterpreted as reflecting the effects of neurological damage rather than the person's attempts to cope with the damage itself.

- Good dementia care should enable people with dementia to display their emotional reactions in whichever way they choose (as long as they are not damaging or hurtful), and should be able to contain and support this emotion.

CHAPTER 10

Managing the Process of Loss

In the previous chapter we outlined the need to understand people with dementia as being caught in a difficult psychological dilemma: whether to block out what is happening to them at the expense of losing touch with reality, or to acknowledge the changes that are occurring, which brings with it an awareness that may be too painful to tolerate.

Since it is our purpose to provide a wide-ranging introduction to dementia, the last chapter – and indeed the one before it – have perhaps made pretty sombre and depressing reading. We have described defence mechanisms which are somewhat dysfunctional ways of staying in control. In this chapter we look at more positive, life-enhancing ways of gaining or regaining control and show how people with dementia are *able* to explore what is happening to them.

Most people with dementia, just like most of the rest of us, struggle to make sense of the world without ignoring the threats that confront them. For people with dementia this struggle is harder because of the magnitude of what is happening to them and also because of the reduction in their cognitive capacity. The challenge with which they are faced is to be able to accept what is happening without losing their sense of uniqueness, of individuality. In other words, they have to be able to hold on to their own identity.

Dementia and identity

So far in this book we have touched several times upon the relationship between identity and dementia. Over the last 20 years or so this relationship has been one of the core concerns of psychologists working with people with dementia. In the psychological literature, dementia has been represented as more than just the loss of particular skills – it has been thought of as involving the destruction of the very essence of what it is to be human: the self. In standard paradigm approaches, this relationship is thought to be a one-way process, with neurological damage leading inexorably to the loss of self. However, the work of Tom Kitwood in particular has broadened this argument so that now it is quite widely recognised that social care practices interact with the process of neurological change to weaken the sufferer's sense of self or personhood.

In Chapter 7 we suggested that many of the psychological and social risk factors for dementia (including occupational status, educational history, age and gender) can be understood in terms of a key variable – the loss of social role. We have argued that it may be the case that such a loss of social roles interacts with the loss of social functioning that results from neurological deterioration. A common factor, then, in social and neurological change is that both may act to reduce a person's involvement with the world around them.

Following a diagnosis of dementia the interaction between internal, neurological change and external, psychosocial change deepens and intensifies. There are at least three ways in which identity is threatened by the onset of dementia.

1. *Directly, through the loss of skills.* As we have described above, dementia is an information processing disability. This compromises a sufferer's cognitive and verbal abilities, and the further the illness progresses the harder it becomes for them to maintain the interactions that are necessary. We have also argued that dementia impacts first of all upon the sufferer's ability to determine meaning and then on their sense of safety. Both of these effects can undermine the dementia sufferer's ability to create and maintain a meaningful account of themselves.

2. *Indirectly, through the loss of social roles.* The diagnosis of dementia carries with it social and psychological baggage: to be diagnosed is to be defined as one of the demented, to enter the shadowy social world of the senile. People with dementia are often assigned a devalued social identity which restricts their lives and the opportunities that are available to them. People around them are likely to begin to react to them differently and will have certain expectations of how they will behave. Often they will be positioned by others within those interactions that are available to them in the devalued role of 'patient'.

3. *The threat of future changes.* The stereotypes about dementia are well known to the sufferers themselves, and the process by which devalued

attributions are made can also turn inward, so that the threat to identity comes not just from the changes in the ways that others react to and define the person but also from the way that the person with dementia views him- or herself. When someone is diagnosed as having dementia, then, even if at that point they are not experiencing many major problems in their life, they may have to rewrite their life script. Their views on their life now and on the life that is to come will change dramatically.

In this chapter we will detail the evidence that we have collected on how someone with dementia responds to or copes with these threats to their identity and the variables that influence this response. However, before we do this we need to outline the view of identity that we will be working with.

Identity

The view of identity, personhood or self that we are using in this book is one in which the individual is seen as actively engaged in creating and holding on to a sense of who he or she is. This model of identity developed from an approach to psychology and philosophy known as the *social constructionist approach*. This approach emphasises that people gain a sense of who they are largely through social interaction – that is to say, our identity is gained mainly from being with other people.

Consequently, a person's identity or a sense of self is not something that can be automatically taken away or destroyed by either neurological deterioration or changes in the social world of the dementia sufferer. Instead, our view is that the person who has been diagnosed as suffering from dementia has to adjust their view of themselves so as to accommodate the changes that have taken place.

This is not to say that the changes that take place within and around a person do not influence them. As we have argued above, the behaviour of people with dementia is often misinterpreted as reflecting the dementing process occurring within the brain. In many cases, however, the things that people with dementia say and do which are frequently thought to be a consequence of the disease can be considered, at least in part, to be a consequence of their attempts to manage the process.

Positioning oneself

One of the key concepts of this approach to identity is that of 'positioning' (McNamee and Gergen 1992). This refers to the way in which each of us takes up or is assigned a particular stance within a social interaction. In acting within a social context we inevitably position ourselves as people who embody certain traits or features. This positioning is integral to our sense of who we are: it concerns our verbal and non-verbal means of telling other people (and ourselves) about the sort of people that we take ourselves to be.

One way to describe the concept of positioning is to use an example that we are probably all familiar with – that of politicians. British politicians, like their counterparts in most other countries, have recently become very adept at presenting a particular view of themselves and their parties to the world at large, often through the employment of specialists or 'spin doctors' who try to ensure that exactly the desired image is presented by journalists. Frequently, the image that a politician wants to present is that of a person who the public can trust to do the right thing. Two of the many means that politicians use to present themselves as trustworthy can illustrate the concept of positioning. The first is the day-to-day political debate and exchange in which politicians engage with their opponents, and the second is the way they describe themselves and their parties in set speeches.

When they are engaged in a debate almost all politicians will employ a series of rhetorical tactics to suggest that their opponents are being unreasonable and untrustworthy. For instance, they may rubbish their political opponents by denigrating their previous record, thus positioning them as people who cannot be trusted. Similarly, they may stress the reasonableness of their own policies or frame their approach to politics as being consistent and based on common sense and that of their opponents as inconsistent and inconsequential. Public discussion of events which might serve to undermine this positioning of themselves as trustworthy is avoided at all costs. Thus, given that most politicians position or market themselves as eminently moral people who support the concept of 'family life', the consequences of having an extra-marital affair and lying about it can be severe. Such behaviour undermines the appearance of trustworthiness that politicians feel that they need to have.

The second way that politicians position themselves is through speeches, newspaper articles and the like, in which there is no tangible enemy to contrast themselves with. In such media they often try to present a history of their policies that stretches back over many years – for instance 'the Conservative Party has always been the party of the family' or 'the Labour Party has always stood for social justice', and so on. The accounts of themselves, their parties and the policies that they represent typically stress certain core values and beliefs. The argument is often made that although their policies may change over time, this is only a matter of their core standards being interpreted afresh for each generation.

Now, in many ways, all of us employ similar devices to provide ourselves with an identity. When we are talking with others, we may chose someone else with whom to contrast ourselves and, just like the politicians, attempt to position ourselves as having certain valued traits or qualities (e.g. 'look, I'm not one of those people who believes in beating about the bush'; 'with me what you see is what you get'). We do a similar thing when we look back over our lives and identify consistency and continuity. When we have behaved in a way that we cannot account for in terms of these core values then we sometimes use special terms such as 'born-again', or 'having a nervous breakdown' to account for this discontinuity.

Identity, in this sense, is not something that we have within ourselves so much as something that we establish through either our interactions with others or maintaining a personal history – which could be seen as an interaction with ourselves. We use social interactions to position ourselves in certain ways.

Coping with a threat to one's identity

For people with dementia, this ability to position oneself in a particular way is threatened by both internal, cognitive changes and changes in social circumstances. The task they are faced with is to acknowledge those changes that have occurred whilst also maintaining a sense of themselves as still being more or less the same person that they used to be. This presents people with dementia with a terrible dilemma: to try to remain the same person without denying that something awful has happened. However, it is difficult to change when this risks conforming to the negative views that others hold about people with dementia.

We can hazard an educated guess at what the successful resolution of this dilemma might involve – namely, the ability to position oneself as someone who, despite the neurological deterioration involved in the illness, has been able to hold on to a sense of themselves as the same person that they have always been. Both within the interactions of people with dementia and within the stories that they tell about themselves, the aim is to be recognised by themselves and others as the same person as before, albeit as someone who now has difficulties.

This process of positioning is not a static one, but rather one in which the dementia sufferer's responses change and develop according to:

- the nature of the loss
- the effect of their cognitive disability
- the social world in which they live.

At first, therefore, it is hardly surprising that many people with dementia tend to respond by using coping strategies that involve shutting out the threat and diverting their attention away from it. Then, as the threat becomes too great to be ignored, the balance shifts and the threat is gradually incorporated into the person's view of him- or herself and the world.

This process of coping is not necessarily one that the person is aware of or can talk about. Although many of the people with dementia with whom we have talked have been able to discuss how they dealt with the problems that they faced, not everybody can be so resilient. People with dementia, like all of us, struggle with life in the best way that they can. In the remainder of this chapter, we will detail some of the ways that people with dementia with whom we have worked appear to have been able to respond to the threat to their identity that dementia poses.

Becoming the person that others take us for

One of the most frequently reported behavioural aspects of dementia is that of sufferers seeming to lose interest in the world. People with dementia are often described as apathetic and lacking in motivation. It is as if they have withdrawn from the world. Often, dementia is even described as a death that leaves the body behind. Such apathy and lack of motivation is often understood in terms of neurological damage to the brain and, in particular, to the frontal areas concerned with motivation and personality. Yet it is becoming increasingly clear that social and personal factors may also be involved.

For people with dementia, the ability to create a sense of who they are – to hold on to their identity by talking and being with others – is compromised in at least three ways. First of all, people with dementia, like many people with an illness, tend to be treated as a collective whole, as if they were all alike. Second, because of the medical approaches to dementia described in earlier chapters, people with dementia are assigned a devalued social identity which restricts their lives and the opportunities available to them. Often people with dementia are seen as not having the same needs as other people and are consequently denied the opportunity to talk meaningfully about their lives with others who have had similar experiences. Finally, the illness itself often robs sufferers of their ability to hold on to a sense of themselves as active, valuable people.

For instance, once someone has been diagnosed as having dementia, people around them will begin to react to them differently and will have certain expectations as to how they will behave. In most cases of persons diagnosed as having dementia, their social interactions do not allow them to maintain a sense of themselves as lovers, helpers, carers, teachers and so on. It is not simply that there is no place for them to perform, even marginally, in these roles, but also that there is no place or permission for them to talk about themselves as occupying these roles. The ultimate result of this situation may be the fencing off of the person with dementia so that they are unable to establish themselves outside these roles, and thus the creation of a self-fulfilling hypothesis (Sabat and Harré 1992). So we should stop saying that the person with dementia is withdrawn and, more accurately, say that their social roles have been withdrawn from them, leaving them only the roles of patient and person with dementia.

It is unsurprising that not every person with dementia is able to hold on to a sense of themselves as a valuable individual. Valerie Sinason (1992), a psychodynamic psychotherapist, has described how people faced with an unbearable situation may defensively exaggerate their difficulties and thus develop a 'secondary handicap' as a defence against the trauma. She suggests that, essentially, when someone is treated like an idiot, then eventually they begin to act like one. The alternative would be too difficult to tolerate, for it would risk alienating those on whom one depends as well as exposing oneself to the painful risk of failure. It is as if the person with dementia shuts out of awareness any knowledge of their experiences in a defensive exaggeration or denial of their difficulties. Awareness of one's own fragility is so unbearable that it has to be thrown away. In throwing away one's awareness one is also throwing away one's intelligence – one is becoming 'stupid' in the literal sense of being too numbed with grief to use one's intelligence. Becoming the person that others take us to be may be an essential means of defending the self against further attack. In ethnological terms, such fulsome compliance should halt the need of aggressors to continue their attack.

What seems to be happening is that not every person with dementia is able to meet the challenge that we have described above. For some people with dementia the views of those around them are so powerful that they are forced to go along passively with them. This enables sufferers to give up struggling against the odds and appease the powerful forces of the institution, yet the consequences for an individual of doing this are severe – they involve being positioned by powerful others in a limited and devalued role.

Some individuals may almost exaggerate the problems that they face for fear of offending those on whom they are dependent. For instance Sabat (1994) reports the case of Mrs R whose observed behaviour at home with her husband differed markedly from that at the day care centre she attended. At home she was said to wander aimlessly, doing nothing or watching television. Her husband cut up her food for her, and reported that she was unable to follow his instructions and did not help in any home-related work. At the day care centre she did not wander unless there was nothing else to occupy her and was extremely helpful to staff and residents. She did not require any help at all to eat and understood instructions well when they were presented in combinations of verbal and gestural cues.

Sabat interpreted the differences in Mrs R's behaviour in terms of the markedly different social care environments that she experienced, suggesting that the clear variations in behaviour occurred in a close relationship with the social setting – where the environment around a person is supportive then they are able to do far more than when the world around them is hostile. It may be that something of this process is involved in what has been described as 'rementia', whereby an individual regains what had been presumed to be lost abilities when he or she moves from an emotionally impoverished care regime to a more validating one.

Moreover, by retreating into themselves and avoiding as much as possible that which is happening around them, some people with dementia may be able to hold on to the hope of normality by avoiding the possibility of failure and avoiding any new challenges.

Keeping up appearances

To say that people with dementia are the objects of stigmatising views is not necessarily the same as saying that these people view themselves in the same way that others see them. Over and over again, in our work in hospitals and nursing homes, we have come across people diagnosed as having dementia whose views of themselves were diametrically different to those of other people around them. Moreover, these people lived their lives according to what they thought they needed – they did not fit into the comfortable staff/patient divide that the staff saw as existing and consequently made life rather awkward for members of staff. In essence, these people insisted on acting as if they were still important people, people of value and worth who should be respected even if they did have some memory problems.

Human beings are social creatures. We all need other people – we are dependent on those around us. One of our social needs is for other people, and especially the important people in our lives, to think well of us, respect us and like us. As a general rule, each of us needs to present an image of ourselves as being 'normal', for want of a better word. Consequently, we try to position ourselves as competent, worthwhile people.

Being able to present the appearance of being normal is vitally important if the person with dementia is to hold on to a sense of themselves as a worthwhile human being. Yet dementia, by its very nature, begins to rob the person with dementia of the appearance of normality. The longer that the illness goes on, the harder it becomes for the person with dementia to present themselves to the important people in their world as still being normal. Moreover, when one cares deeply about other people, it can be devastating to believe that they are worried or upset about one – we try to protect those around us by keeping our uncertainties and fears to ourselves.

Presenting the appearance of being normal in this way is rather different from the strategy of denial that we described in the previous chapter. With denial, the person with dementia suppresses any awareness that they have dementia. The strategy of maintaining appearances, by contrast, is based on an awareness that there is something wrong. What this strategy requires is that the person monitors their own actions so that they present the appearance to others of being all right.

One example of the efforts that people with dementia make to maintain the appearance of normality has been reported by Peach and Duff (1991), who ran a series of support groups for people with dementia. Within these groups there were frequent discussions of the losses that individual group members had suffered, and of the sadness, anger and grief which resulted. Group members were frightened about the diminution of their abilities and some talked of situations in which they had panicked. These people with dementia were able to use the group sessions to unburden themselves of the fears and uncertainties which they had hidden from those around them, and in particular from their nearest and dearest. All were concerned that they should not become a burden on others. Peach and Duff reported that the participants in their group acknowledged:

the considerable effort involved in appearing 'normal' in front of family and friends and in social situations. They do not want others to know how devastated they feel about their memory loss and cover up. (p.4)

The effort involved in this 'cover up' was experienced as exhausting for many group members, who constantly questioned their minds, checking and rechecking themselves. Enormous emotional energy was spent on ensuring that they did not give away any clues as to what was happening inside them. Keady and Nolan found a very similar picture when they interviewed 11 people with dementia (Keady 1997). One person that they interviewed, a 67-year-old man with Alzheimer's disease, described his secretive behaviour and the heightened feelings of tension and anxiety that resulted:

> I knew something was wrong with me, but I didn't want this to be seen by anyone else. I wanted to stay 'normal' but found it was [long pause] hard. A struggle. [pause] I had to make a lot of lists and keep them in the house or car. We argued a lot because I never wanted to go out. Scared you see. I was always terrified that my wife would find out. (Keady 1997, p.29)

One of the most important acts for this man was to try to ensure that his wife did not suspect that he had memory problems. For many people with dementia this struggle to conceal their difficulties is futile. Often the partners themselves notice that something is wrong but, like the person with dementia, keep this knowledge to themselves in order to protect their loved one.

In a similar vein, Sabat *et al.* (1999) have described Dr B, a 68-year-old who had suffered from Alzheimer's disease for four years. Dr B had a Ph.D. and had spent most of his career in the academic world. Now, however, he was unable to drive and could not recall which day of the week it was. According to standard assessment tests he was moderately to severely affected by the illness. Despite, or perhaps because of, these limitations, Dr B took great care to distinguish himself from the other people who attended the day centre. In particular he consistently refused to participate in any activity which he considered a 'filler'. It seemed that Dr B was determined not to be viewed as just another participant in the centre who was defective in one way or another.

By contrast, when Dr B was asked to collaborate by Sabat in his research project, he eagerly accepted. The goal of the work was to try to understand the experience of the Alzheimer's disease sufferer. Dr B began to speak of his work 'on the project' and asked that a sign be put up on a board in the centre to indicate all the times of his meetings.

In this way, Dr B was able to prevent a loss of self-esteem. These interactions allowed him to maintain his sense of who he was; although the existence of Alzheimer's disease was recognised, the views of others as to what was appropriate for a person with this illness were rejected. While it is unclear how the staff of the day centre or his fellow residents viewed this behaviour (although Dr B took care not to offend them) it was his rejection of the conventional behaviour that was expected of him that allowed him to maintain his sense of self and his self-esteem.

Harry – 'My diary is me, it's my life'

One of us (RC) was asked to visit Harry, as his son had become concerned for his well-being. Harry was eighty-three and had lived on his own since his wife died some years before. The house was tidy and apparently well kept. Harry looked healthy but said that he found life very boring and rarely met anyone.

Shortly after RC had arrived at his house Harry produced some handwritten documents which he then pored over. These turned out to be a history of his life, detailing the major events. One entry read simply 'May 13th, 1986. Mary died' and was underlined.

One of the possible therapeutic options open to Harry was that he could join a support group for people who had difficulty with their memory. However, when this was outlined to him, he said that joining the group simply was not an option that he could consider. Harry maintained that he just could not abide being somewhere where other people were not 100 per cent.

It was apparent that Harry was having great difficulty keeping up with the conversation, repeating himself and asking RC the same questions over and over. But Harry said that he felt his memory was as good as anyone else's, and he did not see himself as a person with memory problems. After all, he patiently explained, if he forgot something about his life he could always look at his notes.

Harry said that he had always been someone who kept his life neat and tidy. In the past he had tried not to get too upset when tragedy occurred – he joked that he had been brought up to keep a stiff upper lip. He had first found that it was useful to keep a note of what was happening in his life way back when he started work as a clerk, and gradually his note taking had increased. These notes, he told RC, waving the pages gently in front of himself, were more than just reminders of what had happened: they were himself, they were what he was, they were his life.

The task of the person with dementia, then, is to position themselves within relationships in a way that allows them to assert a continuity with the past and to continue to be seen as the person that they have been. By creating positions for themselves within the world that are consistent with valued aspects of their lives, people with dementia can create an identity for themselves which can accommodate the existence of the illness without being overwhelmed by it.

Len and Muriel – Coping on his Own

Muriel and Len had just celebrated their golden wedding anniversary when Len's first appointment at the memory clinic came through. Although it was clear that he had problems with his memory, these seemed to be confined to one specific area – that of remembering what had been said to him. Although this created a number of specific problems, for instance in conversation or watching television, the doctors at this time did not feel that the problem was typical of a dementing illness.

Yet Muriel was not reassured – she could see that Len's problems were getting worse despite the doctors' reassurances. Over the last year or so he had also found it hard to remember simple things about the house – where the hoover was kept, for instance. She also felt that Len was hiding from her just how bad things were for him. He seemed to have changed as a person, to have become much more irritable and to be lethargic and unwilling to do the things that he had always enjoyed such as playing golf and taking care of odd jobs about the house. She feared taking him out to the local shopping centre for he had recently wandered away from her and become lost. Now he spent most of the morning in bed, sometimes not rising until midday, which was most unlike his previous self.

Len was also worried. He knew that he could not remember things as he used to and dreaded having friends visit for dinner or even for a quick cup of coffee. He felt anxious about what was happening to him and what the future might hold. Len felt safest when he was doing the things that he always used to do and when Muriel was with him. He began to resent her friends visiting and the time that she spent away from the house, and would be angry if she proposed changes to their lives. At the same time Len also desperately needed to carry on as if life was normal – indeed, he made elaborate plans to visit his brother in Australia, as if embarking upon such an adventure would be the challenge that he needed to prove to himself that he was OK.

continued

Over the next few years Len had many appointments to have further neuropsychological testing and a scan. Even though Muriel was sure that he had grown worse none of these tests could show conclusively what his difficulties were. After some time their psychiatrist suggested that they meet a local clinical psychologist. They found that talking together about their fears was difficult but that it helped to ease them closer together. The psychologist suggested that they keep a diary of the day's events. Len enjoyed doing this – he felt that it helped him to hold on to a sense of what he had been able to do. Muriel also kept him busy, making sure that there was always something for him to do during the morning. Len began to use a relaxation tape to help him to control his anxiety about social engagements. Gradually Len became less depressed and fearful and was able to share his worries with Muriel.

There are many different ways in which people with dementia try to maintain the appearance of normality and competence. Just as Keady's interviewee relied on lists, so other people with dementia need to rely more on the world around them to provide them with cues as to what to do. For instance, some people need to have a predictable and regular structure to their lives – to have things the way that they have always been. Changes to this routine (such as attending a day centre or staying within respite care) are bitterly resisted even when a diagnosis has been reached and problems have been openly acknowledged. Keeping things the way that they have always been allows the person with dementia to hold on to a sense of routine and therefore of security.

Creating a new identity: the importance of storytelling

As their memory problem deepens, so it may become harder for the person with dementia to maintain the appearance of normality. Nevertheless, it is still possible to act in a way that accentuates aspects of one's identity that one values, such as being a carer or teacher. This strategy can be clearly seen in the stories that people with dementia tell (Berzonsky 1990; Viney 1993).

Each of us has the capacity to tell many different stories about ourselves and it is partly by these means that we are able to create an identity for ourselves. This autobiography, if you like, is continually updated – it is part of our sense of who we are, what we see as important and what sort of person we take ourselves to be. As our lives change so our autobiography needs to be updated, perhaps with previous events interpreted afresh in line with the changes that have occurred. When our autobiography cannot accommodate these changes we experience psychological discomfort at the discontinuity – we become anxious, afraid, sad and depressed.

The life story of a person with dementia will have to accommodate the changes within them and in the world around them that the dementia brings. They will have to accommodate not only the loss of cognitive abilities but also the membership of a stigmatised social group.

An example of the important role of storytelling has been described by one of us (Cheston 1996) as occurring in a psychotherapy group for people with dementia that he and two colleagues ran. A recurring theme throughout the different sessions was of group members' 'usefulness' in the past. For all of them, there was a time when they were self-reliant, independent people. Group members explained that they had worked as nurses and teachers and had cared for their own children. Seeing their lives in this way created a sense of interdependency rather than dependency – that, placed within a framework of 70 or 80 years, we are all dependent upon each other, upon a sense of social community. For instance, one group member, Daphne, talked of a time during the war when she had nursed an airman who had lost his memory just as others cared for her now. She commented 'I tell myself that God's rewarding me now for what I did during the war days.' Daphne believed that remembering this time in the past helped her to make sense out of her life and said 'now I understand what he went through'.

One aspect of this universal telling of stories about the past is that it can help people to make sense out of their current experiences by making links with their past. This is a process by which what may begin as raw, unintelligible, present-day happenings are transformed into intelligible events which are similar to past challenges that were met and overcome. When we listen to people with dementia we can see that this process of sense-making occurs and that it takes place within the stories that they tell.

Often what happens when someone tells a story is that the story that they tell is in some way similar to experiences that the person is now having to deal with. Essentially, what is happening is that the person is saying 'this is a bit like the time when…'. Telling a story in this way allows the person with dementia to explore some of the experiences of dementia. For instance, one member of a psychotherapy group that one of us (RC) worked with recounted how he had been a pilot flying an aircraft in and out of a jungle.

The landing strip had to be repeatedly cleared as the jungle continually grew back. The narrator used this story as an illustration of how events from the past helped him in the present day when he came across similar situations, although he knew that there was no possibility of a literal similarity (i.e. flying an aircraft). In many ways the remembered past and the present day seem to be metaphorically similar. That is to say, there were aspects of this man's experience of dementia that seemed to him to be similar to finding his way in and out of the jungle (Cheston 1996).

Similarly, Crisp (1995) has described some of the stories that her mother told her as having an added metaphorical dimension. At the stage when her mother was most acutely aware of losing her grip on past memories she spoke several times of how she had been wandering about in the hills, searching for lost fragments of her own mother's tapestry because they meant so much to her. Later she told the story of 'Willy the sheep', in which the central and most elaborate scene was of Willy's peaceful death, surrounded by loved ones, before the symptoms of a dreadful disease make themselves felt. Crisp suggests that it is not difficult to see this as a metaphor for or a mediation on the 'good death' that one hopes will be one's lot and that of those we care for.

Another example of this use of metaphors as a way of making sense of one's experiences has been provided by Unterbach (1994), who described a man with Alzheimer's disease who repeatedly asserted that 'the plumbers are on strike'. Replacing the words 'the plumbers' with 'my plumbing' allowed an enterprising nurse to request a urological examination which subsequently indicated a urinary tract infection. Unterbach reminds us that the need to communicate persists although the ability to do so effectively may decline. Thus, both actions and speech need to be interpreted as indicating a metaphorical as well as a literal need.

If we start from the position of listening to what people with dementia have to say about their world and viewing such talk as one way in which they are trying to make sense out of their experiences, then it is but a short step towards realising that talking about the past or saying apparently bizarre things such as 'the plumbers are on strike' are forms of communication. Indeed, this is such a self-evident thing to write that it should need no justification or elaboration at all. Unfortunately, all too often, people with dementia are not listened to, and what they have to say is seen as meaningless. In this way, when a person with dementia paces up and down a ward, it can be termed 'wandering', with no thought given to what the person might be trying to do by behaving in this way. For instance, Jones (1995) reports the case of Mr G, an 82-year-old retired teacher diagnosed as suffering from multi-infarct dementia. Mr G began to call the staff nurse who was looking after him by the name of his dead wife, something which the staff there referred to as a pseudodelusion arising from a misperception of his visual world. As Jones began to offer Mr G psychotherapy, so it emerged that he was lonely and grieving for his wife. Mr G was able to make use of this form of work until late in the course of his dementia.

This is why the new culture of dementia care has involved a recognition that so-called problem behaviours should be viewed, primarily, as attempts at communication (Stokes and Goudie 1990; Kitwood 1996). Effective comm-unication depends upon more than just the intactness of cognitive capacity; it requires listeners to have both creativity and insight – the ability to make empathic leaps into the communicative frame of people with dementia (Sinason 1992; Sutton 1997). It requires the willingness to listen and to be moved by what you hear. John Killick's poems (1997) based on the words and ideas of people with dementia in nursing homes are very striking evidence for the validity of this approach.

Positioning oneself in this way also allows the people with dementia to hold on to a sense of themselves as people of value in the face of what may be seen as the stigmatising views of those around them.

Dilys – 'I never expected it to be like this'

Stories can also be told about the present and the immediate past – as the example of Dilys shows.

Dilys was an eighty-three-year-old retired village schoolteacher. She had spent much of her life attending to the needs of those around her, first as a teacher and mother and then as a grandmother and voluntary worker. Dilys was admitted to an assessment ward for people with dementia in a severe state of physical malnutrition and discomfort. She was taking nine different forms of medication and her community psychiatric nurse was concerned that she was doing this haphazardly as well as refusing to eat the meals that were delivered to her.

At first, on the ward, Dilys seemed to be in a severe state of cognitive impairment, but as she received a revised schedule of medication and benefited from the regular diet she began to change both physically and mentally. Dilys changed from being amongst the most severely disabled patients on the ward to being amongst the most able.

continued

As she changed physically, so Dilys's behaviour also changed and she began to busy herself throughout the day with helping the more severely cognitively impaired individuals with daily tasks such as eating and going to the toilet. She also attempted to join staff meetings and visited the staff room, where she looked through patient files and records. Dilys's behaviour created tensions amongst the staff group: some were supportive of her apparent wish to be helpful whilst others resented her actions, accusing her of trying to be like them and not knowing her place.

When one of us met her Dilys was able to tell the story of how she had come to be in the assessment unit. She was greatly concerned not for herself but for her son, who was now living in a group home. Dilys was brutally honest about her own life; the phrase 'I never thought I would come to this' was especially poignant for her and she repeated it several times to herself. She was also able to speak about the devastation to her life that her memory problems had caused, about how living on the ward was like being in a prison that she could not get out of, and about how her requests to go home were refused, ignored or trivialised.

Dilys's behaviour seemed to be a means of creating an identity for herself that was separate from those around her and which contrasted with that which some of the staff expected her to fulfil. Dilys was reconstructing her assigned identity by distancing herself from the other patients with dementia and instead aligning herself with the staff. Dilys did not deny that she had dementia, and was able to comment on the awful state that she had got herself into, but clearly differentiated herself from 'those poor dears' on the ward. At the same time she clearly saw her work on the ward as a continuation of her previous pattern of living. What she saw as maintaining her identity as a carer and helper was viewed by some staff as her becoming 'too big for her boots'.

Creating a shared sense of being

Reminiscence enables individuals to both create some sense of meaning out of their experiences and remind themselves and others that they have been more than just a person with dementia. The telling of stories within a group setting also enables individuals to establish a shared sense of who they are. Buchanan and Middleton (1995), for instance, have suggested that talk about the past within a group setting such as a reminiscence group helps to create a sense of shared identity in a number of different ways:

- *Contrasting the past and the present.* When they talk about the past people with dementia often tell of periods during which they were important people or part of valued social groupings; they may have been a nanny to a Lord and Lady, a troubleshooter for Shell or a midshipman on an ocean-going steamer. These identities contrast starkly with their present status as devalued members of a day hospital, a nursing home, or an in-patient ward.

- *Creating a shared identity within the group.* People with dementia often refer to themselves in a way that stresses their age. Together, they seem to represent themselves as 'elders', the possessors of shared experiences of the war, rationing, parenthood and so on. These stories contrast the sufferers in a positive way with the members of staff who, because they are younger, have not had the same wealth of experiences.

Laura Sutton (1997) has referred to people with dementia as survivors rather than victims – people who have survived a lifetime of challenges, and who now need to be understood in the context of their whole lives and given the opportunity to see themselves in this light. As Roy, another member of the group that RC ran, commented:

> You get the occasional period when you can't be helped with anything at all, and you just stop feeling useful. And they [memories] come along almost automatically, they're almost bound to because you can't think of anything else. It's not all life.

For Roy, it was important for him to say that his present life is not all of his life – that he has done many other things and been many people other than the one who sits in the group. Roy seems to be saying at this point that his sense of not being useful is counterbalanced by his ability to reconstruct a past in which it was he who was depended upon by others, and in which he was, indeed, useful.

- *Being able to tell a story is to be put in a position of power.* Telling one's own story and having others listen to it places the storyteller in a position of power (Viney 1993). Storytellers tend to take a starring role within the story itself (Crisp 1995). Stories can be structured around solving a problem or of being of help to others, or they may involve a struggle to overcome great forces. Storytelling is a way in which we can tell others about who we have been and about who we still are. This may well be especially important for people with dementia, who have to struggle not just with the loss of cognitive abilities but also with a much reduced role in the world. Both of these losses threaten their sense of self – their sense of who they are.

As Jane Crisp has written:

> ...at a time when memory is being eroded and one's sense of who and where one is falling apart, narrative provides a means of bringing the fragments together and constructing an active identity for the narrator. (p.137)

Storytelling is not the only way in which people with dementia are able to create and hold on to positive identities. Sensitive care practices that allow the person with dementia to act in many different ways, to care for others, to listen to others, to be the boss and so on, all are important in allowing the person to maintain a sense of their own self-worth.

We will return to this point in Part Three, in which we will argue that there needs to be a much greater awareness of the importance of listening empathically and carefully to what the person with dementia tells us. We will argue that communicating with people with dementia requires the listener to try to enter their subjective world. When people listen sensitively and carefully in this way, and feed back to the person concerned something of what they have understood, then, as we have seen, the person with dementia can feel that they have been listened to and understood, and that they were and still are of value.

Summary of main points

- People with dementia strive to make sense out of their experiences without at the same time losing a sense of themselves as worthwhile and valuable human beings.
- However, people with dementia not only have to deal with the losses that have already occurred but also the threat of future losses to come. Their ability to cope with loss is compromised by both a reduced cognitive capacity and the changes in their social world which restrict their opportunities to receive emotional support.
- Many people with dementia are able to hold on to a positive identity for themselves either by maintaining the appearance of being normal or by accentuating a part of their lives that fits in with an existing way of viewing themselves positively.

- An important part of this process is provided by storytelling. The telling of stories to an appreciative audience allows people with dementia to make sense of what is happening to them, create a sense of continuity with the past and create a shared sense of social being.

- However, when there is strong social pressure to do so, the person with dementia may begin to act in the way that others expect them to do, for instance by withdrawing from the world.

- Often it is impossible to distinguish between behaviour that arises from neurological deterioration and behaviour which is part of the person's attempt to cope with their illness. When considering the causes of such behaviour it is preferable to give the benefit of the doubt to the person with dementia and thus view it as a response to the threat of their illness. This decision should be seen as part of the therapeutic process. It is to the therapeutic processes through which we try to be of aid and of use to people with dementia that we turn in Part Three.

Applying the Person-focused Approach to Psychological Interventions and Services for People who have Dementia

CHAPTER 11

Psychological Interventions
An Introduction and Basic Principles

In the first part of this book we outlined 'the standard paradigm'. In many respects, this framework remains the most dominant view of dementia within our society. In standard paradigm approaches dementia is seen almost exclusively as a disease of the brain – a process in which neurological integrity is lost, causing both cognitive and behavioural changes. As a result of the dominance of this perspective the emphasis of dementia care has tended to be on maintaining the person's physical health, while their subjective experiences have been, if not completely disregarded, then certainly seen as not being of central importance. The consequences of this neglect of the subjective have been severe in terms of the quality of care that has been available to dementia sufferers.

In the second part of this book we proposed that in psychological terms dementia can be best thought of as a process that erodes an individual's sense of security. This insecurity arises from many sources, including the loss of cognitive abilities, the loss of social roles and social opportunities, and the threat of further losses to come. This erosion of inner security can be so severe that many of the non-cognitive symptoms of dementia such as wandering and denial can be thought of as having their origins in the dementia sufferer's responses to the process of dementia. We described this developing approach to understanding the process of dementia as a 'person-focused' one.

What we want to do in the remaining chapters of this book is to begin to look at the implications for services to people with dementia of this emerging new approach. We can break this down into two main goals:

1. To increase emotional security.

2. To create and maintain self-worth and a sense of identity.

There are many ways in which these goals can be reached. Table 11.1 outlines some of them. You will probably be able to think of other ways.

These approaches should influence dementia care *from the point that an initial assessment is being discussed right through to the dementia sufferer's death.* In the next chapter we will look at how the process of assessment can act to intimidate the people being assessed and contribute to their anxieties and fears, reinforcing their sense of themselves as being unable to operate as they used to do. We will then outline how we believe assessment for ?dementia should be framed, understood and undertaken.

In Chapter 13 we will outline how we can help dementia sufferers to deal with the insecurity and the emotional load of having dementia, while in Chapter 14 we will examine how we can design services to help the person with dementia to keep hold of a sense of him- or herself as someone of value – a sense of identity. Finally, we will turn our attention to the broader issues of service delivery to help people with dementia continue to live in the community, and consider methods of changing the nature of services through teaching and evaluation.

We fully appreciate that the forms of caring that we and others have suggested are asking a lot of carers in that they require them to make sustained emotional contact with the people that they are caring for. We know that this is something that many carers already do. But we also know that wherever people with dementia are cared for their care-givers, be they relatives, voluntary workers or professional health or social service staff, also feel overworked and undervalued. How then can we expect people who are already giving everything that they have to give more?

The answer is that we cannot – not without changes to the system. A person-focused pattern of care can only emerge when embedded institutional practices begin to change. It is not enough to appeal to carers and nurses themselves – dementia care desperately needs more resources and, almost as importantly, a shift in the way that dementia is viewed. This requires organisational change, and it is this issue that we will address in our final chapters.

Table 11.1 Therapeutic interventions aimed at helping to establish 1) emotional security and 2) a consistent sense of identity

Goal 1: Achieving emotional security

Target method	Examples
See emotional needs as of primary importance	Offer long-term support from the beginning of interventions
	Provide support groups for people recently diagnosed as having dementia
Recognise attachment needs	Facilitate maintenance of loving relationships between relatives and sufferers
	Explore the possibility of using simulated Presence Therapy (See Chapter 13)
Minimise catastrophising	Explain that assessment will be to ascertain specific problems (not 'global losses') and that therapy will be available to help with them
	Set up regular individual counselling
Maximise stability of environment	No 'respite care' outside home *or* respite only in familiar surroundings
	All services needed throughout treatment available in person's home locality
Maximise interpersonal stability	Person to be helped by a small team of staff with a high skill quotient and a low staff turnover ('Keywork team')
Minimise stress in person's system	Optimise communication between person and important others. Monitor and minimise stress levels of important others through carer support and input into family
	Provide carer education and training
Minimise random events and extraneous noise	Control noxious aspects of the environment
Create conditions to increase likelihood of above	Provide care within small, well-designed units that maximise orientation, continuity and interpersonal familiarity

Table 11.1 continued

Goal 2. Creating a consistent sense of identity

Allow grieving for losses	Initiate individual counselling with staff skilled in handling losses and grief
Teach problem solving	Use problem-solving approach, maximising client agency and environmental controls
Encourage new friendships	Look at ways of providing day care which encourages people to interact
Encourage the development of emotional support	Look at establishing groupwork drawing on common experiences to encourage group cohesion and networking outside the group
Re-expanding the social network	Attempt to establish contact with old friends, for example, through the Church or British Legion
Reverse internalisation of unemployment uselessness	Encourage expansion and enjoyment of retired role
Maximise esteem-creating activities	e.g. Help client to use long-term memories to teach schoolchildren about the past
Reverse dependency	e.g. Encourage client to make gifts, send greeting cards etc. to relatives and friends
Increase ease of memorising	Structure sessions to make days memorable through personally meaningful events, outings etc.
Encourage new learning or re-learning	Establish 'failure-free teaching' Provide structured outings to previously familiar localities
Minimise disability	Substitute activities to maintain interest (e.g. crocheting or embroidery) Explore the possibility of establishing prosthetics ('dial-a-ride' to get to where you drove previously)

Summary of main points

- Services to people with dementia should be developed around the need to help people to feel more secure and of worth. This involves at least two elements:

    Increasing emotional security and

    Helping people with dementia to maintain a clear sense of their personal and social identity.

- For these goals to be achieved, both a shift in the way dementia is viewed and more organisational resources are required.

CHAPTER 12

The Assessment of People who may have Dementia

A truly person-focused approach to dementia care must attend to the needs of the person with dementia at every point of contact, from first to last. Indeed, assessment is one of the most important areas to ensure that we get right – it sets the tone for what is to come, and if potential problems are not addressed at this point they can become harder and harder to deal with. It is here that we should begin the task of meeting the emotional and identity needs of people with dementia. We can be more succinct: the assessment process must cease to be an end in itself. It must become the beginning of a meeting of the person with a problem or problems with another person who is focused on trying to help them with their problems.

In the first part of the chapter we will describe in detail some of the shortcomings of current assessment procedures. In the second part we will describe the elements that we feel make for a person-focused approach to assessment.

Neuropsychological tests

Neuropsychological assessments are a familiar feature of the services for people with dementia – they are an integral part of the diagnostic procedure. Two sorts of neuropsychological tests are in use:

- General and relatively short screening tests are available for use by almost all qualified mental health professionals. Three of the better known screening tests are the Mini-Mental State Examination (MMSE) (Folstein *et al.* 1975), the Clifton Assessment Procedures for the Elderly (CAPE) (Pattie and Gilleard 1979) and the Middlesex

Elderly Assessment of Mental State (MEAMS) (Golding 1988). For a review of the screening measures see Twining (1991).

- Screening assessments attempt to provide a brief measure of a person's general levels of functioning. However, because they are pretty inexact, people who are thought to have dementia are increasingly being referred to specialist services known as 'memory clinics', where far more detailed neuropsychological tests can be carried out.

If the initial screening test is unclear and the clinician is unsure as to the cause of a person's problems, then more sophisticated and lengthier tests may be used. These tests provide a structured means of assessing a person's cognitive abilities and disabilities. A person's results on these tests can be compared with the results that would be expected from healthy people of the same age. These assessments, of course, take longer, perhaps several hours, to complete.

Neuropsychological assessments are in no way emotionally neutral for the person being assessed. Rather, they can have profound effects on the patient who has to go through them. We will now spend some time considering what these effects might be before suggesting some ways of countering the more damaging aspects of them.

Limitations of neuropsychological assessment

Shoham and Neuschatz have commented:

> The most disturbing factor, however, was that there seemed to be a demeaning element in the constant memory testing. It was obvious that the procedure was painful to many of the patients who could not manage to recall the information asked for. The authors felt that the constant reminder of the patients' failure of memory served to reinforce their sense of inadequacy. In a population in which individuals frequently laughed at the sometimes grotesque errors of their peers, this procedure seemed to have a strongly anti-therapeutic element. The authors found that other observers have come to similar conclusions.
>
> Because memory is so basic to human functioning, it is understandable that memory loss has traditionally been identified as the primary problem of senile individuals. In an institution, however, nursing staff enable patients to function without the patients having to depend totally on memory. The authors concluded that there were other aspects of the patients' sense of self that were more devastating than loss of memory. Humans are essentially social beings who need to interact with

others. They need to communicate. An individual's self-image feeds in
good part on how he or she is seen by others; positive feedback is needed
to be able to survive and flourish. (Shoham and Neuschatz 1985, p.69)

An interesting although somewhat disturbing feature of psychometric testing is that very little attention is paid to either the social context of the testing
situation or the impact of testing upon individuals. The emphasis in training
clinical psychologists or student mental health nurses to use these tests, for
example, tends to be on the importance of administrating and scoring
psychometric tests correctly ('reliably') and not on the likely impact of these
tests on patients. (We refer to the person being assessed as 'the patient'. In our
opinion, the label 'patient' best reflects the sociology of testing in that testing
is done to or on a person and there is an inherent power differential
underpinning the formal assessment procedure.)

   We believe that the impact of psychometric assessments can be seen as
falling into a number of areas of concern.

TESTING AND ANXIETY AND DEPRESSION

Testing does not occur unless problems have been reported by the patient or,
as is more likely, by the people around him or her. The patient, then, may well
have high levels of anxiety and depression before the testing begins and it is
likely that the process of being assessed will create further tension and
anxiety. We can see the emotional side of dementia as a downward spiral in
which the feelings of anxiety, threat, depression and grief that we described
in Part Two are all likely to be involved (see Figure 12.1).

Possible signs of dementia/early dementia
▼
Awareness of loss
▼
Help-seeking
▼
Anxiety as various assessments are undertaken
▼
Awareness of losses as various assessments are undertaken
▼
Loss of self-esteem/depressed mood
▼
**Lowered mood and anxiety further add
to decreased intellectual and memory functioning**
▼
Person believes/accepts diagnosis
▼
Further awareness of losses
▼
**Further increase in anxiety at undertaking tasks;
further increase in depressed mood**
▼
Etc.

Figure 12.1 Anxiety–depression spiral concerning assumed dementia
Note: This flow diagram has similarities with that of Kitwood (1990a)

DIFFERENCES IN POWER AND STATUS

The patient role, by definition, is a position of lower power and prestige than that of the assessor. Being in the presence of a person of greater power will often act to increase the individual's uncertainty and anxiety. These relationship features can be accentuated if, as is likely, the patient perceives leaving the interaction 'prematurely' as involving heavy penalties. 'Upsetting the doctor' or their colleague is rarely considered a useful or profitable strategy, and therefore the patient could be considered as being imprisoned within the assessment situation: unable to leave but unwilling to continue.

Furthermore, as the majority of seriously ill patients and those diagnosed as 'psychotic' are likely to be poorly educated and from the lower socio-economic classes (Hollingshead and Redlich 1958; Littlewood and Lipsedge 1989), there is also a class imbalance. There is, therefore, a clash of different verbal and non-verbal behaviours. It is hard to envisage how, in such circumstances, the patient could ever feel in control of the situation.

The sense of lack of control is important, for the implications of a poor test result for a patient can be profound: for instance, having their driving licence removed, having to consider giving up work or, at another extreme, having to consider admission to residential care. For many patients, then, the process of neuropsychological testing accentuates into their fears of dependency and incompetence, producing a sense of anxiety and threat. For those being assessed the implications are very frightening and it is crucial, therefore, that the emotional and social contexts of assessment are understood and addressed by the person conducting the test.

NOT UNDERSTANDING WHAT IS GOING ON

Most patients are not told in detail why they are being assessed. Generally, the assessor may give some vague, bland explanation as to the real aims of the assessment, perhaps mentioning concerns about memory, finding out how you're getting on and so on. In our experience it is comparatively rare for patients to be told that the reason that they are being assessed is to see whether or not they suffer from dementia. For the patient this leaves a number of questions unanswered, such as: 'What is the assessor's expertise?' 'What does Dr X actually want from me?' 'What are the implications to me of this assessment?' The patient may also wonder what phrases such as 'How are you getting on?' or 'How are you feeling in yourself?' actually mean.

In most assessment situations, then, the first task for the patient is to decide what the test is measuring. The assessor may have given them a full explanation, a partial explanation or a 'cover', i.e. a benignly inaccurate explanation. We would hypothesise that few people believe these explanations and instead reach their own conclusions. Thus, the first stage is the search for what the test 'is getting at'. We can illustrate this process by providing some quotations from a study by John Keady and Mike Bender on people with early onset dementia:

> 'They kept putting me in a room and asking me to do all these things ... counting and things. I never knew why I had to do it and I didn't want to go back. I got frightened and worried because I knew I couldn't do what they wanted.'

Male spouse with very mild dementia, aged 67 years

and

> 'I never knew what to expect. I didn't want to go but she [patient's wife]
> made me. What were these things for? I did what they wanted me to and
> sometimes I didn't because I [pause] didn't want to look stupid.'
>
> Male spouse with very mild dementia, aged 74 years (Keady and Bender
> 1998, pp137–138)

Any attempts by the patient to clarify the purpose of the assessment are likely
to be met with further platitudes. However, it is more likely that the assessor,
through their verbal and non-verbal behaviour, will indicate that commenting upon and questioning the assessment procedure is not welcome. Thus,
not only are the purposes of the assessment nebulous and confusing, but this
nebulous confusion cannot be talked about.

Given these circumstances it is likely that patients will usually believe that
only one or two traits are being measured. Having decided what it is they are
being assessed on, the second stage of the process is to decide what stance
they wish to take. This will be influenced by the information the assessor is
asking for and the implicit knowledge that this information will be shared
amongst those people close to the assessor. For instance:

> 'I never trusted anybody there [the memory clinic]. I knew something
> was wrong with me and they were trying to find out what, but I was so, er,
> scared. I thought everyone would know if I failed something. I never
> wanted to fail anything but I knew I did and I think they knew it too.'
>
> Female spouse with very mild dementia – aged 72 years (Keady and
> Bender 1998, p.138)

The third stage of the process involves the patient positioning themselves in a
way that allows them to gain some control of the situation. Thus, if the
patient decides that the questionnaire is measuring depression they will then
decide how 'depressed' they wish to be during the assessment. If they are on
a psychiatric assessment ward and wish to stay there they may well wish to
give the impression of being 'very depressed' and will fill in the questionnaire in that direction. If they would prefer to go home they may well present
themselves as 'not depressed'. Thus, they are working out the payoffs for
various stances. The process is shown in Figure 12.2.

Stage One	Brief, benign explanation of purpose of assessment given with implication that patient should *not* seek clarification
	▼
Stage Two	Patient decides what traits are being measured (accuracy of this understanding is irrelevant)
	▼
Stage Three	Patient decides how they wish to present themselves with regard to these traits
	▼
Stage Four	Patient fills in the form in the way that most accurately, to their mind, presents this self
	▼
Stage Five	Experimenter scores answers as if tests are measuring an absolute value

Figure 12.2 Decision tree of a person filling in a questionnaire

Note that the accuracy of the patient's understanding of the inventor's purpose in designing the form – what the test inventor thinks it is measuring – is quite irrelevant. If the patient decides that 'I sweat easily' is a measure of virility or 'I hear voices' is a measure of acuity of hearing then this is the basis on which they will proceed to Stage Three.

This model, in effect, relates the process of being assessed to the notion of positioning that we outlined in Part Two. The patient is deciding what position to adopt with regard to what they think is being measured. While it may be possible to refuse to answer questions, this is a difficult position to maintain because of the risks involved in upsetting the powerful and losing access to treatment. In addition, patients are often required to answer a series of questions which, in many cases, seem to be unrelated to the memory or cognitive problems that they may be experiencing. At times, the content of the questions can seem childish or patronising. Moreover, in most neuropsychological tests the questions become harder and harder until the patient either gives up or provides the wrong answer. The experience of repeated failure can thus compound a person's sense of themselves as incompetent.

By participating in the assessment the patient risks being positioned in a way that is inimical to their often fragile sense of being a person of worth. As Tom Kitwood has suggested, these assessments can be intimidating and consequently form part of the malignant social psychology that so often surrounds people with dementia.

THE SOCIAL CONTEXT OF MEMORY ASSESSMENT

As we have described above, the most common and simple to use neuropsychological assessments are the screening tests. These screening measures attempt to ascertain, in part, a person's orientation to time, place and person – which is, more or less, the working definition of disorientation used by most clinicians. There is an expectation that the person being assessed should be oriented to the time of day and the month, and be able to recall where they are, their own name and the names of famous people such as the Prime Minister.

In part, however, this process of orientation relies on social context. When people are assessed as being disoriented, therefore, this may reflect as much a dislocation in their social context as it does a decline in their cognitive abilities. We will illustrate this argument by looking at some of these markers.

Common questions in the screening measures include asking a person if they can remember the day of the week, date and season. The assumption behind this line of questioning is that a normally competent person knows all of this information without recourse to their diary, calendar or other aid. However, normally competent people do *not* rely solely upon their memories to answer such questions, especially if it is a matter of any importance. Rather, we use external aids to prompt our recall: diaries, calendars and so on, and most importantly of all, event markers. What we mean by this is that we know it is Monday, for instance, as it is the first day at work after a weekend (this accounts for the common experience after a Bank Holiday Monday of being mildly disorientated as to the day).

The normally competent older person is even more likely to lead a life in which time is divided up by various types of different events. For example, Monday might be washing day, Tuesday keep-fit day and so on. Here, life has markers as to the day. A life which has fewer or no such markers such as life in an unstimulating environment, be it in a person's own home or in an institution, invites disorientation. The person in such a situation is not disorientated in time. Rather, we would suggest, *they are not orientated to time by events*. But a memory assessment takes no account of such a social context – it makes the categorical assumption that a person who is disoriented in time is likely to have a cognitive deficit and discounts as irrelevant the possibility (or reality) of an impoverished social environment.

Just as screening assessments ask the patient for the day and the date, so they also frequently require patients to recall where they are. Yet one of the features of psychological assessment is that it often takes place away from the patient's home in an assessment/rehabilitation ward many miles away. Therefore, the frequency with which the patient has visited the place where the assessment is conducted is low and, by extension, their ignorance of its name is likely to be higher. Once again, the interpretation of the available evidence in terms of cognitive deterioration is compromised by the social context.

Therefore, the present measures of memory risk confusing the ability to memorise with the patient's level of social engagement. (Interestingly, the patient may make this connection by stating that they have lost interest in what year it is, but this behaviour is then construed as evidence of either depression or a defence against actual memory loss; either way, its credibility as a satisfactory explanation is discounted.)

The person-focused approach to assessment

Although over the last ten years or so the emphasis within dementia care has shifted away from understanding dementia simply in terms of brain functioning, the culture of testing has hardly changed at all. This cannot be allowed to continue: assessment procedures need to be guided by a philosophy of care that places the emotional and social needs of the dementia sufferer at the forefront of clinical work. We would like to suggest that a clear set of guidelines would help to establish a person-focused form of neuropsychological assessment. Table 12.1 lists the ways in which we believe the assessment procedures for ?dementia[1] must change.

Taking each point in table 12.1 in turn:

1. *Assessment is the first step in a long-term collaborative relationship between the professional worker and the person with dementia.*

One reason that the relationship between assessor and patient is so fraught and ambiguous is that it is so hurried and so truncated. The relationship

---

1   ?dementia refers to those people who believe they have, or are believed by others to have the early symptoms of dementia. This may or may not be so.

between the assessor and the patient is seen as a means to an end, rather than as something that could be therapeutic.

On occasion, where the difficulties are due to remediable physical or psychological causes – urinary tract infection, pneumonia, stress etc. – this shortness of the assessment relationship may be acceptable; but clearly, a Memory Clinic is in business to 'find' and then assess people with dementia (often for the main purpose of enrolling them within drug trials) (Bender 1996a; Moniz-Cook and Woods 1997). Such people will usually show declining skills with time, with correspondingly greater need for services. Therefore, the service should be geared to forming and maintaining a long-term relationship with them.

Table 12.1 Main aspects of a person-focused assessment for ?dementia

1. Assessment is the first step in a long-term, collaborative relationship.

2. Assessment only occurs after informed consent has been obtained.

3. Assessments focus on living in the community.

4. Assessments are undertaken in the person's home and community.

5. The person being assessed is informed that they will receive full feedback after the assessment is complete and when this will happen.

6. The assessment places the person within the context of their whole life; and examines how any possible disabilities relate to the person's life history.

7. Assessments do not merely gain evidence for diagnostic purposesbut focus on specific difficulties.

8. The person's emotions and beliefs about their problems are also part of the assessment.

9. The person should be assessed within the context of their interpersonal and family situation.

10. The person being assessed is able to control who else receives the results of the assessment.

11. Feedback of the assessment, including diagnosis, occurs sensitively and with an empathic understanding of the person's emotional world.

12. The results of the assessment are provided in an understandable written statement as well as given verbally.

13. Services are offered straight away, not only after a crisis has occured.

14. Services are offered independently of whether drug therapy will be started or not.

At present, people with memory problems are often assessed as to the cause of such memory problems at a point where they do not yet have the sort of difficulties that require additional input from the mental health or social services. Once a diagnosis has been provided, these people are then, essentially, left to their own devices until their cognitive state has deteriorated to such an extent that an intervention is thought to be appropriate.

This simply isn't good enough! It really is outrageous that dementia sufferers and their families are left to deal with the implications of an (often unreliable) diagnosis without any support. Both sufferers and their families should be given as much practical and emotional support as possible after the assessment has been carried out – for instance in the form of support groups to help them to prepare and to think about the future.

This problem stems from an essential flaw in most services – they view assessment as something that is entirely separate from intervention. Yet, as we have argued here, assessment is not a neutral activity – it comes at a sensitive time in people's lives and can make a large emotional impact. If dementia services are to become person-focused, then assessments must be seen as the first part of establishing a relationship between the person suspected of having dementia and the people who provide the services to support them.

If, for reasons of lack of finance or other resources, no such care can be offered to people in these early stages, then what on earth is the point of doing the assessment in the first place? If the assessment does not lead on to a qualitatively different form of care and support, then, as mental health professionals, we really have no business doing an assessment at all.

In this light, the first task of the assessor, as team member, is to form a relationship of trust with the person with dementia; and this key task should last as long as it takes to achieve its goal. In creating trust, the person who is thought to have dementia has plenty of time and opportunity to start seeing the assessor as a helpful and trustworthy colleague in the cooperative venture of finding out what is happening to them; and taking the risk of being less defensive, and more aware of the benefits of being in control of their life.

2.   *Assessment only occurs after informed consent has been obtained*

A fundamental plank of medical ethics is that no medical intervention (and this includes assessment procedures) should proceed without the patient giving 'informed consent' to it. In terms of neuropsychological assessments, we cannot consider that meaningful consent has been given to the assessment unless such consent is based on an informed understanding of the purpose of the assessment. Thus, patients who are referred for neuropsychological assessments should routinely be given information as to the reason why such tests are being considered. They should be told, for example, that the doctor wishes to assess whether they suffer from a depressive illness, or a global organic deficit such as Alzheimer's disease. Where necessary, the patient should be offered pre-testing counselling before a decision is made as to whether or not they will take part in the testing (as is the case with testing for HIV or AIDS).

Although, at times, it may be necessary to invest a considerable amount of time in talking through the possible consequences of the test with the patient before even starting the procedure of testing, working in this way is likely to result in both much more reliable test results and also a more efficient and effective way of helping people tackle emotional problems later on. As one 69-year-old patient from a study by Keady, in Keady and Bender (1998), revealed:

> I wanted to have more say and information on what was happening to me. I never knew what was going on most of the time. I felt a little used to tell you the truth.

3. *Assessments are about helping the person stay in the community*

We are, of course, aware of physical and interpersonal situations which make it dangerous for the person to stay in their home, whatever the level of service provided. It may also be the case that, on occasion, the person wishes to leave their home. However, we wish to redress the present balance whereby assessment is often used to prove that the person requires care. So, by focusing on the goal of community living, we seek to offer assessment early on in terms of cognitive losses; and we aim to specify the skills and interpersonal factors that may put their community living at risk; and thereafter provide the range and depth of services to minimise that risk. In short, we work within the framework of dementia as a disability affecting community living.

4. *It follows, then, that the only logical place to offer and undertake functional assessment is in the person's home.*

The setting in which an assessment occurs is important. It may well be more appropriate that physical examinations be done in a surgery than in the home; and that cognitive assessments should occur in a local office where quiet and freedom from intrusion can be more certainly achieved. Such examinations can be undertaken in the person's GP surgery, so that there is no need for hospital visits.

However, when it comes to practical skills, one of the absurdities of the present scene is that people with dementia are often admitted as in-patients for assessment. As part of their assessment they may well be asked to prepare a meal to assess their ability to cook for themselves. The person, already anxious at being asked to undertake the assessment, is then given a different set of utensils and equipment, in a completely different location and layout.

No wonder they perform poorly. Functionally we might argue that the purpose of such units is to deliver the throughput of 'people with dementia' that the local dementia service requires for its maintenance.

We are aware that a person may be more resistant to doing an ADL (Activities of Daily Living) assessment in their own home. But then, the whole philosophy we are proposing is that assessment has to be the beginning of a cooperative venture; and this philosophy has a knock-on effect on the relationship between the person with dementia and their important others. By establishing a lasting relationship, we can begin to help the person with dementia and those around them to begin to adjust to the problems they face. A person can usually maintain that everything is alright only if people around them go along with them. We need to move to services which, with their person-focus, acknowledge the views and rights of both the person with dementia and of the others in their familial system. And we need to start this process by assessing the person in their own environment.

5.   *The person being assessed is informed that they will receive full feedback of the results of the assessment and when this will be.*

A person being assessed must be guaranteed: 1) as much feedback as they wish; and 2) a specific session at which this feedback will occur. It is possible, of course, that they do not wish for feedback. We would not see this wish as a static constant but one that may change as the assessment proceeds and as the relationship of trust between assessor and patient, hopefully, deepens. Therefore, the patient's wishes regarding feedback can be re-checked at a time nearer the allotted feedback slot.

(If the initial lack of interest in feedback led to the cancellation of the feedback interview, this would be unfortunate as it might be some time before it could be re-scheduled, which is clearly undesirable.)

6. *The emphasis of assessment should move away from a concern with diagnosis to take account of the person within the context of their whole life.*

Assessment techniques need to become more user-friendly, to focus on the person in the round, and to take account of the person's unique biographical history and social situation. The Gloucester project headed by Malcolm Johnson (Dant *et al.* 1989), for instance, described both a personalised approach to assessment which involved taking a full biography and basing the provision of services around this extended context. They found that such an approach made a considerable difference. It is essential, therefore, that a full life history and the person's narrative of it is gathered during the assessment; and that the test results are understood in the light of that life.

7. *To examine the level of functioning and disability.*

Neuropsychological assessments do not just provide results to firm up a psychiatric diagnosis – these tests should also examine the areas in which the person is particularly deficient or disabled, as well as detailing the effects of those disabilities on the skills of the person. Such a functional assessment would look at the nature of the skills lost and possible remedies, and their self-perception.

Holden (1995) provides a similar approach: if we make a more functional assessment of a person's difficulties, then we will be much more focused on what their actual difficulties are. We also then increase our chances of being able to design effective interventions (Emerson and Frampton 1995).

8. *To ascertain the person's emotions and beliefs about their problems*

We need to be aware, not only of the nature of the impairment, but of the person's reaction to it. This includes the patient's previous level of security and coping skills, and their past history. We have already discussed Bowlby's attachment theory (Chapter 7) which would predict that present styles of handling difficulties will be crucially determined by the quality of a person's early relationships.

9. *To gain an understanding of their interpersonal and family situation.*

The interactions within the patient's family and other systems that they live in are also clearly vitally important to understand, as the person re-negotiates their position and standing in the light of their difficulties and devaluation.

10. *The person being assessed is able to control who else receives the results of the assessment*

We start with two very basic principles, that we see affecting all interactions between the mental health professionals and the person who is being assessed for ?dementia, and their relative.

The person with ?dementia – the patient – is the person who has the right to feedback and the right to specify who receives that feedback. We would suggest that, at the moment, the primary relationship between dementia workers, such as in memory clinics, is not between professionals and patient but between professionals and relatives. (In many ways, it is similar to the situation in the field of learning disabilities.)

Recently, clinical psychologists have moved towards giving the client their diagnosis; but, implicitly, this is within a framework of the client being seen with the relative. We are advocating that the client be seen first to discuss whether they wish the relatives to be informed – a reversal of current practice. We are saying that the information belongs to the client. Therefore, the decision whether or not others have access to that information is theirs to make.

We are aware of the great difficulties that such a position creates if the person who is ? dementia is in denial of their difficulties and might refuse an assessment based on an honest explanation of its purpose.

However, we would suggest that such a position may encourage greater honesty within the family and, therefore, this denial mode may become unsustainable.

With dementia, there is no escape from pain; but we can be almost certain that a relationship between assessor (and their colleagues) and the patient that starts out based on subterfuge and deliberate confusion is most unlikely to develop into a relationship of trust.

So, for a while, we do agree that there will be difficulties in developing an approach where the client controls information. But remember: the client controls the dissemination of information in the case of diagnoses such as cancer or AIDs where a professional would be liable to reprimand, if not worse, if they divulged personal information to others without the patient's consent. We are also aware that this primacy of the doctor–relative relationship, rather than the doctor-patient relationship, is endemic in the field of the care of the elderly. But, again, that is no reason why people with dementia should not be extended the same courtesies and rights as people with almost any other illness.

11. *Feedback of the assessment, including diagnosis, must occur sensitively and with an empathic understanding.*

In some ways the phrase 'breaking bad news' is something of a misnomer. At least in the early stages of dementia, most patients are already aware (at some level) of something being wrong and of others acting towards them in new, and unusual, ways. Also, disclosing a diagnosis should not mean that patients or their relatives will be forced to confront issues that are too emotionally loaded for them to deal with. Rather, it places the emphasis on patients and carers exploring these important issues at their own pace.

While counselling people with dementia is in the early stages of development, there is a much more established body of literature concerning the 'breaking of bad news' in palliative care. The main features of this approach include:

- providing sufficient time for individuals to explore the meaning and implications of the diagnosis
- *if desired* having a relative or carer present during the initial discussions of the diagnosis
- providing sufficient information at the right time in ways that are easy for the patient and his or her family to access
- encouraging the acceptance of emotional distress while allowing the possibility of hope to exist.

While we have stressed the primacy of the wishes of the person with dementia to determine what is fed back to them, there are many people, including professionals, who feel that the relative(s) have the right to specify the degree, if any, of feedback to the sufferer. Therefore, if this issue is not clarified at the beginning, then there can often be a very tortuous negotiation between the relative who wants to know but who demands that his or her husband or wife is not told, and the clinician who wishes for a more complete disclosure to the patient.

12. *The results of the assessment should be provided in an understandable written statement, in addition to the verbal feedback*

It is well established that patients take in only a limited percentage of what professionals such as GPs tell them (Ley 1982); which is not surprising given their level of anxiety. How much more must this be the case when you are getting feedback as to whether you have a chronic, deteriorating brain disease!

Written information should be provided so that the patient and their carer can consult it later on. A follow-up session or a contact number should be provided, so that the patient does not feel that they have been abandoned. These are very simple suggestions, but it is unfortunately the case that there are still many assessors who present information in a one-off way that can be very distressing.

So, written feedback should supplement the interview. Perhaps a videotape with illustrations and diagrams explaining the person's specific difficulties might be even more useful. Yet another possibility is that a video of the feedback session is given to the person to take away with them.

13. Services are offered straight away, not only after a crisis has occured

At the beginning of this section, we said that the assessment had to be the beginning of a long-term relationship. Here we reiterate and expand this point.

Even if the diagnosis is of possible dementia and the prognosis 'merely' of possible problems in the future, this news may be quite devastating for the person; and seriously decrease their ability to cope and function. Their reactions after they leave the assessment cannot be predicted from how they behaved when they were getting the feedback. For example, their 'acceptance' may have been a response of shock and denial. Also, any feedback may radically change the familial dynamics. So, accessible, professional services must be offered after any assessment for ? dementia independent of the outcome; and services resourced accordingly.

14. Services must be offered independently of whether drug therapy will be started or not

The emotional reactions of receiving a diagnosis will not conveniently go away, just because the person receives a prescription. So, whether they get put on a drug or not should in no way affect the mental health services they require and receive. They don't stop being a person because they get some possibly – but probably not – efficacious drug. And no drug can take away the fear and terror that comes with a diagnosis of dementia; and therefore cannot take away the need for skilled mental health input.

The effectiveness of the psychologists and others involved in providing this diagnostic service, often within a memory clinic, should be regularly assessed by finding out the satisfaction of patients and their carers with the service that the memory clinic has provided.

Conclusions

We have given assessment considerable attention as it appears to highlight many of the deficiencies of existing services, and because we wish to position it as the necessary beginning of a longer-term relationship.

Policy makers and service providers need to develop ways of responding more fully to the lived experience of people with mild dementia, their family supporters and their social networks. The depth and breadth of investment which will be necessary to operationalise this process should not be underestimated. There is an urgent need for more openness and honesty. We need the voices and experiences of people with dementia to become a foundation for dementia care practice and service planning.

The provision of a proactive early dementia service needs to be based upon the availability of resources and specific targeting, coupled with a willingness to communicate diagnoses and, perhaps even more importantly, prognoses. This openness hinges on identification and individualised assessment of specific problems, which require an intimate understanding of the social and biographical context in which such problems are occurring.

Summary of main points

- A truly person-focused service has to be comprehensive, covering all aspects of service delivery beginning with the moment that a referral to a specialist service is made.
- There should be no assessment without informed consent.
- Assessment should focus on keeping the person in the community if that is their wish.
- Functional assessment should take place in the person's home.
- Neuropsychological assessments are often intimidating and distressing events for people who are being assessed. A series of changes needs to be made, beginning with the person concerned and their family being offered pre-assessment counselling and an ongoing, long-term, supportive relationship. Approaching assessments in this way may also minimise tensions that may arise later on in the procedure.

- Where testing occurs, this needs to be placed within the context of a wider range of assessments and a focused approach to actual difficulties. The person's concerns about their future and their need to maintain their own identity should be at the forefront. Assessment should be the start of a therapeutic relationship, not a brief, unsatisfying, frustrating encounter.

- Testing should also lead on to further support and intervention. It should never be the case that assessment becomes a goal in itself, divorced from practical help.

- We outline a set of specific guidelines for achieving the goal of integrating assessment as the beginning of a long-term, collaborative relationship.

- These guidelines show the need for a radical reorientation of the role of assessment within the services for people with dementia.

CHAPTER 13

Therapeutic Interventions

Maximising Self-security – The Vital Role of Listening Skills

In the second part of this book we described how, in psychological terms, dementia could be seen as a process in which a person's sense of inner security comes under attack. This attack takes the form of fundamental changes in the dementia sufferer's information processing capacity and skills, creating a great sense of emotional turmoil and a potential threat to the dementia sufferer's ability to maintain a sense of who they are.

In the introductory chapter to this part of the book, Chapter 11, we introduced two major types of therapeutic needs of people with dementia – those of emotional security and the maintenance of personal and social identity. The second need – identity maintenance – is more likely to be the therapist's major concern when dealing with people with mild/moderate dementia; but the therapist will not succeed in their endeavours unless and until they have reassured the person that they are secure with them. Indeed, it is almost certain that *no* therapy, regardless of the person's abilities, can be undertaken until the person feels safe. You cannot work on a person's identity – or rearrange their Meaning System – until you have managed to get the alarm switched off.

So, before we engage in identity maintenance, we must satisfy the need for security. We will address this area first. The achievement of emotional security is a major therapeutic goal *from mild to very severe dementia.* It is a worthwhile therapeutic task in its own right. It legitimises therapeutic work with the very cognitively damaged, and calls for the development of many approaches, especially ones that are less verbally dependent, or non-verbal.

So, the achievement of security is both a prerequisite for verbal therapies and, more importantly, a major task in itself for all people with dementia.

We think feeling safe is crucial where there is cognitive loss, and that this achievement of security has to be a central concern of all types of services for people with dementia. It is particularly vital when cognitive deficits are more severe.

Emotional security comes from many sources – from routine, from familiarity and, in particular, from having close confiding and supportive relationships. In this chapter we will explore how the ability to create such relationships through the use of good listening skills is an essential part of good dementia care.

It is only possible to feel emotionally secure when one's closest personal relationships support such security. It is not possible for any of us to feel emotionally secure over a sustained period of time if these relationships are destructive. Emotional security, then, is partly a product of how people relate to us. Therefore, in services for people with dementia, the key determinant of the quality of care that clients receive is the personal interaction between clients and staff. Where a client receives good quality care, then in many cases there may not even be a need for further interventions – their emotional and identity needs will already have been met. We need to consider, then, the basic ingredients of good interpersonal relationships – the abilities to listen and to communicate to others that they have been listened to and understood.

Maximising felt security: the vital role of listening skills

At the heart of good quality dementia care is personal contact which is guided by an empathic awareness of the experiences of the dementia sufferer. As Ian Morton has pointed out:

> ...when we are concerned with people with dementia, there is no other way of working that will meet the most fundamental need for genuine human contact, acceptance and warmth ... Partners, family, friends, nursing staff, care staff and the other people with whom the person with dementia spends a significant proportion of each day are the only potential 'treatment' that we have to offer. (Morton 1997, p.372)

It is through the provision of such sensitive interpersonal care that emotional change becomes possible. This care requires the use of listening and other skills in an informal manner as part of the task of relating to the person with dementia. We are not talking here about *doing formal* psychotherapy with dementia sufferers individually or in a group. The issue that we want to emphasise here is one of *being* psychotherapeutic in dementia care. By this we mean *the importance of using every interaction with the person*, whether this be to offer a cup of tea or to accompany them on a walk to the toilet, *as a potential opportunity to help and to support them.*

1. The need to bear witness

We said earlier that much of the behaviour of those health and social care professionals that people with dementia meet (such as the extended assessments or the frequent failure to offer emotional support and nurturance to the people with dementia themselves) can perhaps be usefully understood as the behaviour of people who cannot refuse to interact with people with dementia but who wish to avoid contamination. This behaviour means that there are few safe places in which the person with dementia can explore this process and begin to make sense of what is happening to them.

Consequently, one of the most important aspects of using listening skills with someone with dementia is to enable that person to feel that their experience of dementia is important. This can help to provide a context of care in which the dementia sufferer feels valued, which can in turn help to promote within them a sense that the process of loss can be tolerated. In order to bear witness we need to stay (in an emotional sense) with what people with dementia tell us about themselves and provide them with the space and time to do this.

It is important, too, to bear witness over a period of time. As dementia creates enormous uncertainties and fears for dementia sufferers, it is important that there should be some figures who are always present, reassuring and familiar.

2. Empathic listening

Empathic listening involves attending not only to the content of what a person is saying and whether it is factually true or not, but also to the emotional themes and messages that lie beneath the surface message. These skills are most often associated with humanistic, especially Rogerian, counselling (Rogers 1961, 1978; Rogers and Stevens 1971; Thorne 1992). One of the most influential uses of Rogerian counselling skills in work with people with dementia has been Resolution Therapy (Goudie and Stokes 1989; Stokes and Goudie 1990). Resolution Therapy encourages carers to empathise with the hidden meanings and feelings which are thought to lie behind the confusion expressed by people with dementia.

Stokes and Goudie described much of the confused behaviour and talk of people with dementia as resulting from attempts to make sense out of the world – attempts that are hindered by the dementia sufferers' cognitive deficits. Stokes and Goudie claimed that provided tentative reflections and acknowledgements of the dementia sufferer's feelings are accurate and delivered with sensitivity and patience, the person's feelings begin to become clearer and the reasons behind apparently 'confused' behaviours begin to emerge.

Being able to express such deeply-held emotions may have a cathartic effect. That is to say, it may help to release pent-up feelings. Although this is potentially painful it is also vital if the person with dementia is to be able to make progress. The acceptance of emotional distress resulting from these losses is not just an issue for the person with dementia – their relatives may also have much emotional work to do and little opportunity to acknowledge or own their feelings.

Effective dementia care, then, depends upon effective communication, and effective communication requires listeners to have both creativity and insight – the ability to make empathic leaps into the internal world of people with dementia. It requires the willingness to listen and to be moved by what you hear and to communicate your understanding back in a form that the other person finds acceptable. Thus, within good dementia care environments, the interactions between residents and between residents and staff can be marked by a whole range of behaviours, from praising and complimenting through to gentle, humorous mocking of self (Frank 1995) (though not, of course, mocking of another).

3. Listen to the whole message

As social animals we all use many forms of communication, of which only one is language. We need, then, to pay attention to the facial expressions of dementia sufferers, the way that they hold their bodies and so on. Often this takes the form of attending to the person's rhythmical rocking or to the way in which their hands fret and play. At these times a non-verbal reassuring response, such as gently stroking the person's hair or shoulders to relax them may be appropriate. It is also important to listen for subtle changes in the way that the person speaks such as slight changes in tone (Morrow, Allen and Campbell 1997).

4. Listening to the metaphors that people use

As we described in Part Two, the language and stories that people with dementia tell often involve themes of loss: lost friends and family members; threats that have been overcome; and of problems that have been successfully resolved. By attending to the thematic meaning of the language used by dementia sufferers rather than being distracted by its literal content we may be able to understand much more.

The task of the carer in this context is to give the person with dementia the sense that they have been listened to and that what they have said is of value and importance. Communicating with people with dementia requires that the listener tries to enter into the subjective world of the dementia sufferer – into their communicative frame. As Tom Kitwood (1990b) suggests:

> We need to slow down our thought processes, to become inwardly quiet, and to have a kind of poetic awareness: that is to look for the significance of metaphor and allusion rather than to pursue meaning with a kind of relentless tunnel vision … The crucial issue is not that of adjusting the dementia sufferer to our everyday reality, but of adjusting ourselves or 'tuning in', to his or her emotional reality. (p.51)

When people listen sensitively and carefully in this way, and feed back to the person concerned something of what they have understood, then the dementia sufferer can feel that they have been listened to and understood. When he or she is struggling to cope with the process of dementia then such empathic listening and responding may be psychotherapeutic, for instance facilitating a process of emotional change or perhaps even of grieving.

5. Being aware of the differing needs of the patient and their relatives

To understand the context of their work, professionals need to be highly sensitive to the fact that relatives and patients can be angry, overprotective, very anxious about themselves and each other. But the needs of patients and relatives are not synonymous. In fact, we would go further and say they *rarely* are. It is unlikely that their meaning frames, hopes, fears, wishes or desired solutions are identical – however much each may assume they are – if only because they are different people facing a very difficult situation. So, we need to be person-focused and recognise the subjectivity of the person with dementia *and* the subjectivity of their relative. Of course, balancing the needs of carers and dementia sufferers can be extremely difficult, for instance when a relative asks that the person with dementia should not be informed of the diagnosis or of decisions that have been made. If we aim to build our service around the needs of people who have dementia then the decision should always be made in favour of disclosure to the patient unless there are strong reasons to the contrary.

6. Being aware of the unspoken needs and wishes of the professionals

Just as we have to separate the needs and wishes of patients and relatives, so we must not misidentify professional rhetoric as altruistic, scientifically-based wisdom. We need services that are clearly based around patient needs, not service needs. For instance, nobody that we have met ever needed to attend a day hospital. Attendance at a day hospital was the response of the service to the person's need to overcome social isolation, anxiety, depression, and so on – needs that for *some* were met at the day hospital that they attended.

7. Understanding the person's life history

We can never hope to fully understand an individual unless we are aware of their life history. Yet standard psychiatric assessments of people with dementia often contain little that can help us to achieve such an understanding. In particular, we need to find out more about any losses that they have suffered in the past and their methods of coping with stress – in short, to learn more about them and their life as they lived it.

We are therefore recommending that counselling be available to all people with dementia. A small pilot project, the Companions Club, offering such regular support throughout the 'career' of the person with dementia is described in Bender *et al.* (1999). A more comprehensive and integrated service has been established at a Day Hospital in Gala (see Box 3.1).

By 'counselling' we do not just mean being sympathetic to the plight of the other! It is also important that the problem-solving focus discussed in the last chapter with regard to assessment is maintained. This is one technique, among others, that helps to prevent 'catastrophising' (Ellis 1962; Beck 1976).

Beck defines 'catastrophising' as 'In any situation in which there is any possibility of an unpleasant outcome, the patient dwells on the most extreme negative consequences conceivable' (p.154). Nowadays, perhaps, we talk of the person imagining (and believing in) the 'worst-case scenario'. Clearly,

---

Box 13.1 The Gala day unit

As a way of illustrating the role of psychotherapy within a clinical environment, we will describe some of the issues set out in two recent papers in the *Journal of Dementia Care* (Moyes and Christie 1998a; 1998b), which describe how psychotherapeutic skills were employed in a day unit at Gala in the Scottish borders.

Within the day unit the daily routine of activities and groups was flexible enough to allow individual support and therapy sessions with members of staff, who are experienced in counselling skills as well as mutual support groups. This was achieved through a creative use of the limited amount of room space available, so that both individual and group sessions could be available.

The effect of this structured but informal counselling can be seen in one day unit client whose cognitive state was deteriorating quickly. This man was able to tell a member of staff about his concerns: he was aware that others saw him as being hopeless and he had resigned himself to becoming so dependent that he would need hospital admission. The day hospital staff decided on a structured plan of support and counselling from the day unit staff. The client gradually came to recognise and accept those areas in his life in which he could not manage independently. His family were also encouraged to focus on his feelings and abilities as opposed to his diagnosis. From having been depressed with a strong sense of hopelessness, the man gradually began to emerge as a confident and happy person who had much higher levels of self-esteem and could be assertive, both about his own needs and those of another person, a frail elderly lady at the day unit.

---

with such a framing of present and future events, the person will feel terribly insecure. So, through our individual and groupwork, we need to strive to limit the (very real) problems and make them manageable, and maintain the person's belief in their ability to retain (some) control of events.

What we are trying to do is to move from the client's *global* feelings of worthlessness and hopelessness to a consideration of *specific* problems and how they may be overcome (Heider 1958; Bender 1998).

Many of the more specific ways of achieving security were outlined in Table 11.1. Rather than elaborate upon that list, we will now use attachment theory to provide a rationale and a framework.

Maintaining secure attachments

As we described in Chapter 8, one of the most influential frames within which the experiences of dementia sufferers has been placed is that of attachment theory. Not only does this theory place the experience of the dementia sufferer within the context of a well-articulated theory of emotional development across the lifespan, but it also opens the way towards developing a range of new interventions. To recap:

Attachment

This term refers to a set of concepts initially set out by psychoanalysts such as Bowlby (e.g. Bowlby 1972) and extended by developmental psychologists including Ainsworth (e.g. Ainsworth *et al.* 1978) to explain the behaviour of very young children in terms of their relationships with their parents. Once an attachment has been established (generally to the parents and especially to the mother) the infant tends to cry when they are separated and show pleasure when their attachment figure returns. Moreover, at times of stress, for instance in a strange situation, the infant will seek out their attachment figure and gain emotional reassurance from their presence. The child's efforts to search for and cling on to their attachment figures are described as 'attachment behaviours'.

Attachment and dementia

Many dementia sufferers face the disruption of their attachment relationships as the decline in their cognitive abilities makes it harder for them to 'hold on to' their attachment figures when they are not physically present. The frequent provision of respite and other services which separate the sufferer from their main carer may also disrupt these attachment relationships.

Research is only just beginning on how we can help people with dementia to maintain strong attachment relationships. Clearly, the most effective way to do this is to provide support within the community so as to enable the dementia sufferer to continue to live with their relative for as long as possible. Where the person with dementia lives on their own the main attachment may well be to material possessions, and a sense of security may be created simply by being within their home.

All too often respite care does the opposite of what it intends. Rather than *maintaining* the bond between the relative and the person with dementia it *weakens* it. The respite care removes the person with dementia to a place which is unfamiliar to them, causing spatial disorientation and loss of skills (as many skills are no longer applicable in the strange new environment). Respite care, in many if not most cases, engenders strong feelings – whether verbalised or not – of abandonment and betrayal. The person who returns home is emotionally more frail and has to re-learn their old skills – an extremely difficult task for a person with dementia. So their level of functioning is further reduced, and their ability to use their skills is damaged by their feelings of insecurity – feelings which, from an objective point of view, are very rational. The relative quickly loses any benefit they might have gained from the break. The greater stress of the relationship quickly leads to a request for a further respite…

In short, respite care gradually breaks the resolve of the relative to care for their loved one by presenting increasingly difficult tasks to an increasingly exhausted person. Figure 13.1 presents this diagrammatically.

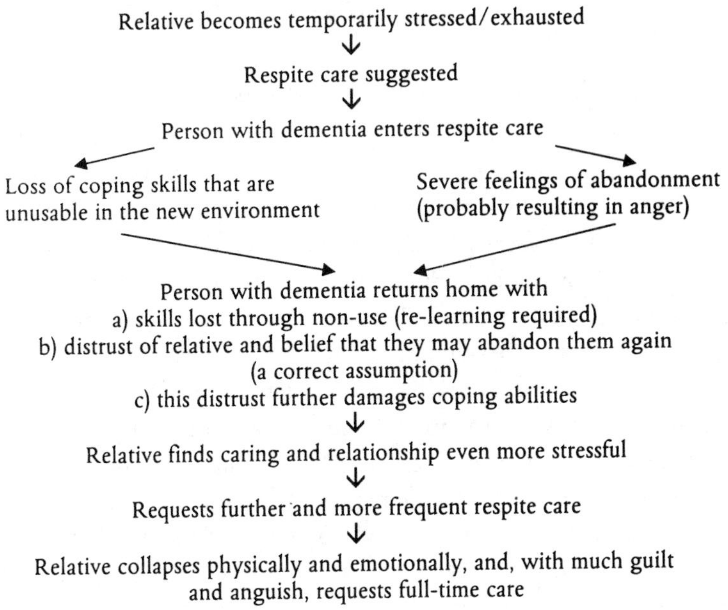

Relative becomes temporarily stressed/exhausted
↓
Respite care suggested
↓
Person with dementia enters respite care

Loss of coping skills that are
unusable in the new environment

Severe feelings of abandonment
(probably resulting in anger)

Person with dementia returns home with
a) skills lost through non-use (re-learning required)
b) distrust of relative and belief that they may abandon them again
(a correct assumption)
c) this distrust further damages coping abilities
↓
Relative finds caring and relationship even more stressful
↓
Requests further and more frequent respite care
↓
Relative collapses physically and emotionally, and, with much guilt
and anguish, requests full-time care

Figure 13.1 Respite care as the functional route to the breakdown of the maintenance of the relationship between a person with dementia and their caring relative

It is for these reasons that, in Table 11.1, we advocated *minimising loss of familiar surroundings* if a respite break is needed by the relative. (It was for the same reasons that, in Chapter 12, we advocated functional assessments being undertaken in the home.) If possible, this means the person with dementia should stay in their own home, supported – at the needed level of intensity – by familiar staff such as home care. If, understandably, the relative does not want a holiday away and would rather stay in their own home, respite might be provided within the unit providing day care. So, the professional organisation of the respite should proceed along the path of choosing the option that minimises unfamiliarity.

We know that, even when support is provided, it just is not possible for every person with dementia to live out their life within the community. Yet placing someone in a strange environment with people that they do not know will almost certainly increase their insecurity, leading to more attachment behaviour. In such cases there are several ways in which we can try and help dementia sufferers to hold on to those existing attachment figures in their lives:

MAINTAIN EXISTING ATTACHMENT RELATIONSHIPS

All too often, when a dementia sufferer is admitted to a home or hospital, the role of their relative changes out of all recognition, often to the distress of both the relative and the dementia sufferer. The relative moves from a position of having the person with dementia almost completely dependent on them to one in which they are not only separated physically but also often excluded from the practice and planning of care. Both the relative and the person with dementia are often devastated by this change.

We need to be aware of the tensions between the relative who has cared to the point of exhaustion for their loved one and the admitting nurse or residential worker. The relative, perhaps feeling that they should have held on for a little longer, may see little improvement in the quality of care their spouse/parent is receiving, and indeed may see a decline. This viewpoint, of course, implicitly criticises the unit's staff. The admitting staff, on the other hand, have to believe that they have greater competence than the carer – otherwise, what use were their years of training? This attitude implicitly criticises the carer.

If the admission is handled badly – as seems all too often the case – the staff communicate to the relative – implicitly or explicitly – that they will be undertaking all the care needs from now on, leaving the relative no role. In this way, the inevitable tension is handled, but handled badly and at a terrible cost to the relative's well-being and their relationship with the person who has dementia, just at a time when the attachment bond is most needed.

Good dementia care practices recognise the benefit of the relative continuing to provide as much care as possible. After all, it was not so long ago that children's wards refused to allow the parents of even very young children to stay with them during their hospitalisation – a practice that is now universally seen as callous and uncaring. The same thing needs to happen within dementia care. Health and social services should actively provide a variety of services – joint carer and patient units, halfway houses and so on – capable of meeting the varied attachment needs of couples and architecturally equipped to cater for greater physical dependency, thus dispensing with the need for relocation. It is cruel and degrading to expect couples who may have been married for 50, 60 or even more years to have to separate because they have become too frail to continue to care physically for each other.

ESTABLISHING NEW ATTACHMENT RELATIONSHIPS

Many good and emotionally sustaining relationships are established between people with dementia and nurses, health care workers and care assistants. When such relationships occur they can help to ease the blow for dementia sufferers of losing their primary attachment figures. It is as if a new attachment relationship is being established.

We also know that many more such relationships could and should be created. There are at least two reasons why they are not more frequent. The first is due to attitudes amongst care staff and the second is organisational. The first reason that more relationships are not established is because, by and large, they are not seen as fundamental to good care. In many units it is still the case that only physical care is valued, and talking to the patient is seen as an irrelevance ('they don't understand') and a waste of time. Also, in some units there is a belief that close relationships between nurses and their patients can lead to 'burnout' amongst health care staff and are therefore discouraged. This is based on a misconception: cynicism and burnout are caused, we believe, not by having close relationships but by having relationships with patients (close or otherwise) that are not supported or recognised by others as being important. The infrequency of such relationships is also partly due to the standard paradigm view of people with dementia as diseased brains – and we can only have relationships with people, not with brains, diseased or otherwise.

The second reason why more close relationships do not occur is organisational. Again, there are many factors that operate to discourage such relationships, from low levels of staff to the use of unpredictable shift working. One of the most important reasons, however, is that those care assistants and health care workers who have the highest levels of patient contact (and who therefore have the most chance to develop meaningful relationships with them) are the least trained.

They often are very caring but 1) have little control over their professional lives, and so often cannot provide the continuity needed to create security; and 2) because of the lack of interest in training such staff, they are not given any framework that stresses the importance of their relationships with their patients. In all too many units it is made clear to them that such contact is secondary to the need to provide physical care; and, for almost all, the value of their caring is not highlighted and reinforced. Training, in short, could and should provide them with a structure and approach that encourages and consolidates their efforts to include and maximise respect for their patients; and, by giving their posts more prestige, would give such interactions legitimacy and value.

TRANSITIONAL OBJECTS

It is vital to help the dementia sufferer to carry with them into their new setting as many familiar things as possible from their old setting, and thus help them to feel emotionally secure. Just as young children who go to a nursery can feel comforted by their favourite teddy bear, so elderly people with dementia may feel comforted and reassured by having with them some familiar objects. These 'transitional objects' have some of the qualities of the attachment figure and can ease the child (or in this case the person with dementia) through a separation from their attachment figure. For older people, transitional objects can take the form of photographs, cats, favourite items of clothing, treasured mugs and so on.

All too often, when visiting clients in residential and nursing homes, we are struck by the acres of empty wall and shelf space crying out to be filled by mementoes and symbols of the life they lived and the people they knew and know. It is no wonder that in such surroundings they have often been referred to psychology for depression.

SIMULATED PRESENCE THERAPY

One intervention that attempts to provide people in residential care with a familiar, emotionally reassuring presence is Simulated Presence Therapy (SPT). This was the name given by Woods and Ashley (1995) to a technique that they developed in which dementia sufferers living in nursing homes were played a tape made by their care-giver on a personal stereo.

Mary

Byatt and Cheston have described the case of a sixty-nine-year-old lady, Mary Smith. Despite Mary sometimes being in considerable physical pain from her arthritic hips, staff at the centre were concerned by Mary's wandering, which continued throughout the day. However, when either her husband or daughter visited, Mary's behaviour was very different: she was able to remain seated, eat her meals and express clear enjoyment of their visit, smiling, chatting and using increased amounts of eye contact.

On the first four occasions that the tape was played to her, Mary remained seated whilst listening to it for up to 35 minutes. During this time, Mary also appeared to be more aware of her environment, interacting with others and showing some concern for their welfare, behaviour that was at other times mainly absent. For example, during the first intervention Mary waved to another resident with evident pleasure and laughed at things that she heard on the tape, saying, 'that's lovely', 'he's right isn't he?' and 'that's his niece'.

However, following the fourth session, Mary was suffering levels of pain that clearly interfered with her ability to gain any enjoyment or satisfaction from the memories tape. It was noticeable that during this time Mary also lost much of her ability to draw comfort from the presence of her husband and daughter. As Mary no longer seemed to derive any clear benefit from the tape the intervention was halted.

Two months elapsed before Mary's pain had been reduced by a change in her medication so that she could listen to the tape again. During these sessions Mary seemed once again to become increasingly engaged with and orientated to her environment. Whilst listening to the tape and in the period immediately after listening to the tape, Mary would attempt to either engage others in interactions or join others in their social interactions. For instance, she offered another resident an item from the kitchen area; responded to a question from the occupational therapist who was facilitating a group discussion; received a cuddle from another resident; and apologised for stepping on someone's toes.

While these examples may appear to be rather trivial, for Mary they represented significant changes in her usual behaviour. Staff of the unit commented on Mary's increased well-being, shown in such ways as her being able to feed herself at meal times, relax for limited periods with others and increase initiation of social interaction with both staff and other residents.

Woods and Ashley reported the effects of using such tapes with 36 subjects, finding that the behaviour of 31 of them improved with the use of SPT 'most of the time'. They claimed that there were significant reductions in the amount of both disruptive behaviour and social isolation when these tapes were played. Woods and Ashley interpreted the effectiveness of SPT in terms of helping to lessen the attachment anxiety experienced by dementia sufferers by providing the voice of an adult attachment figure.

This idea of playing tapes to dementia sufferers, therefore, represents one way in which it might be possible to lessen their attachment anxiety. One of us (RC) has been involved in setting up two pilot projects to test out the effectiveness of this intervention (Byatt and Cheston 1999; Cheston and Peak, forthcoming) with dementia sufferers on an in-patient ward.

The use of SPT is at an early stage, but nevertheless it provides one possible means of attempting to meet attachment needs. In many ways the improvements in Mary's behaviour can be taken as an example of a process that has been described as 'rementia' (Kitwood 1996; and Sixsmith, Stilwell and Copeland 1993) in which the dementia sufferer seems to be lifted to the top level of their functioning, performing at a level that had seemed to be lost. Although it is important to recognise the generally high level of nursing care that Mary received, the SPT tape may also have helped her to gain a secure emotional base, enabling her to move from her position of withdrawal into her inner world and engage in a limited way with her environment and those within it.

Some research carried out after this original case study serves as a reminder that the attachment histories of individuals are not the same (Peak 1999). Observation of Mary's behaviour prior to our intervention suggested that she had a secure attachment relationship with her husband, but this will not be true of all dementia sufferers. Peak and Cheston also worked on the same ward with another five sufferers, two of whom, like Mary, seemed to have secure attachments with their spouses. For them, the tapes were once again listened to positively.

The other three patients, however, are probably best described as having either an ambivalent attachment relationship or as being avoidant. For these three, the SPT tapes seemed to be much less effective and in some cases were distressing. (Incidentally, the tape recorder is worn on a pouch around the waist, and its physical presence seems to prevent the belief in disembodied voices coming from the walls!)

So far we have looked at interpersonal relationships. We end by stressing the need for the physical environment to reassure and remain familiar. The person should be helped by a small number of staff who know them well; their routine should not create failure and should allow them to experiment and practise their skills with a low rate of failure experiences; and they should be addressed respectfully and their experiences and opinions should be valued. All such work is rendered valueless if the environment is stressful because there is shouting or crying, people running around, loud, unexpected sounds, or instructions to move or do things without explanation. Yet so often we see staff who understood what they should be doing but do not appreciate the paramount importance of creating an environment which will allow their efforts to succeed. If there is no security there can be no therapeutic success.

As we come to the close of this chapter we want to emphasise that we see routine as a *structure* rather than as repetition. So, by 'routine' we mean that the day has clear markers – 'When I get to the unit I know I will be greeted by Wendy and will have a cup of tea with three other attenders. Then we'll do an activity'. The marked-out day allows for initiative and experimentation within secure and known boundaries.

Feeling secure is an ongoing process. Its achievement allows the staff and the person to tackle the second major area of endeavour – maintaining a valued identity.

We emphasise again that achieving security is very much a goal in its own right. If the person feels secure, the skills and memory deficits caused by anxiety and depression will decrease or even drop away; the person will feel that they can experiment, that they can take and try out advice, and that they do not need to deny or pretend not to be interested. On this foundation, staff can build and encourage greater flexibility and re-learning of old skills. Meeting the need for security will allow for greater use of existing skills and thus a higher level of functioning. Therefore, the creation of security in one-to-one interactions, in the small group, in the home and in the day-to-day running of all units where the person with dementia might go is a vital goal – if not *the* vital goal – in helping people with dementia, regardless of the level of their difficulties.

Summary of main points

- Little can be achieved in work with people who have dementia if such work is not undertaken in an environment in which they feel secure.

- The achievement of security can be facilitated by regular individual counselling, which encourages a move from global devaluation to focused problem-solving and, generally, works to prevent catastrophising.

- If there is a need for respite it should be planned on the basis of minimising loss of familiarity.

- It is important that new clinical interventions are developed which allow people with dementia to hold on to primary attachment figures, encourage them to develop new attachments and recognise the importance of other forms of attachment, including the use of transitional objects.

- Another major aspect of achieving that security is maintaining and encouraging existing social relationships.

- If those relationships cannot be maintained in their home we should encourage and facilitate relationships in the person's new accommodation.

- We should work to create an environment which is free from stress and random, unexplained events.

CHAPTER 14

Identity Work
Holding on to Who We Are

> After all, what is this lump of matter if you can't make sense of it?
>
> [A person with dementia to John Killick], *Killick (1997)*

In the second part of this book we argued that one of the key psychological determinants of dementia is the loss of social role. Dementia, in this sense, can be understood as a process that undermines a person's identity. Those people for whom fewer social roles are available are, consequently, more vulnerable to neurological deterioration, which, in turn, erodes a person's capacity to sustain their remaining social roles.

This process of identity loss is not an automatic process of change, but depends to a very large extent on the psychosocial world that surrounds that person, and, most importantly of all, on the quality of care that they receive. This interaction between social and neurological losses is often compounded by patterns of care which, in many cases, see people with dementia not just as patients but also as people who have lost the ability to reason, to communicate satisfactorily and even to feel – in short, as non-people.

In this chapter we will set out what we believe to be some of the important ways in which we can structure our services so as to enable individuals with dementia to maintain a sense of their own identity. We must allow them to retain a sense of personal continuity – of being the same people that they have always been.

We shall look at psychotherapy with people who have dementia, but we will also look at identity maintenance *throughout the spectrum of cognitive difficulty.* In no way do we want to give the impression that identity work can only be done with the verbally able. The techniques must be modified, but the importance of the task and the need for it stay the same – we all need to feel that we exist as people and that our existence matters.

Identity work

There are many different ideas within psychology and philosophy about what it is that gives each human being a unique psychological make-up. In this book we have used the term 'identity', but as we have seen, Tom Kitwood, for instance, has talked about a slightly different concept, that of 'personhood'.

Whilst there are important conceptual differences between these differing psychological perspectives there is also much that is shared. In particular, there is widespread agreement about the core element that enables people to hold on to a secure sense of being – positive social interaction. It is through our interactions with others, our friendships, our love affairs, our conversations with Uncle Bill, that we become who we are. Take these relationships away, or so distort them that they become constrictive, and each and every one of us will be vulnerable to an erosion of our sense of who we are. For dementia sufferers, who are struggling against an internal process that robs them of verbal and cognitive abilities, the potential damage that can be caused by a restrictive social world is greater still.

We will now discuss three contrasting examples of psychological thinking about identity and use these concepts to provide illustrations of how the form of care that people with dementia receive can help them to retain a secure sense of being.

The three approaches are:

1. The psychodynamic

2. The social constructionist

3. Structuring care to maintain personhood.

Psychodynamic concepts of identity

The psychodynamic perspective draws heavily on the work of Sigmund Freud (e.g. Gay 1988 and Sinason 1992). It views identity as something that is to be found in the internal, unconscious processes to which we are all subject. In particular, the sense of who we are is described as the *ego*. The strength of the ego is in part determined by the person's earliest experiences, but also depends upon other internal and external forces. For a person with dementia, the ego's strength may be compromised by the process of cognitive loss and also by the form and quality of care that they receive.

In psychodynamic terms, it is thought to be possible to slow the process of identity loss by establishing a consistent relationship with others. Although this is often thought of as being a 'therapeutic' relationship, it does not necessarily have to be with a therapist – a caring person can establish such a therapeutic relationship so long as they have sufficient empathy to allow the dementia sufferer to express their emotions openly.

Through their empathic stance, the therapist is able to become a new ego or self for the dementia sufferer, either recognising and validating the client's competencies and capacities or providing a calming, reassuring and supportive presence (O'Connor 1993). Organising the patient's environment so that as much change as possible is avoided and the environment remains constant may also help the dementia sufferer to maintain a secure sense of who they are. Similarly, providing stimulation and encouraging tactile, sensory and affective responses may also strengthen the ego (Unterbach 1994), a point to which we will return later in this chapter.

Psychotherapy with dementia sufferers

In the first part of this book we described how psychotherapists had largely ignored work with people with dementia. We will now outline how psychotherapy skills can be used with dementia sufferers. We will not go into great detail about what the skills of psychotherapy are, as there are plenty of other books that do precisely this and we assume that many of the people reading this book are already familiar with at least some of these techniques. The emphasis in this section will be on how to use the skills that many psychologists, social workers and nurses already possess with this client group.

PLACING PSYCHOTHERAPY WITH DEMENTIA SUFFERERS IN CONTEXT

Although there have been consistent reports of psychotherapeutic work with dementia sufferers stretching back over 40 years (Gilewski 1986), this form of work has failed to make a significant impact until recently. In this respect the United Kingdom seems to have lagged behind continental Europe, and in particular France, where there is a much stronger tradition of psychotherapeutic work with people with dementia. A range of interventions have been used including psychodynamic psychotherapy (e.g. LeGoues 1988; Maisondieu 1995), cognitive psychotherapy (Myers-Arràzola and

Bizzini 1995) and systemic psychotherapy (e.g. Ploton 1990) (see Cheston 1998 for an overview).

The reluctance of psychologists, psychotherapists and others in Britain to engage people with dementia in psychotherapy has been at considerable cost to those they might reasonably have been expected to try to help (see Chapter 5). There are so many points in the 'career' of a person with dementia at which a therapeutic space for them to spend time thinking about what has happened or challenging their catastrophic thoughts would be of benefit. This is true from the point of diagnosis through to admission to residential or nursing home and beyond.

We argued in Chapter 5 that therapists had largely ignored working with older people in general, let alone people with dementia. Yet convincing clinical evidence is beginning to accumulate which suggests that such work is not only possible but can also be extremely beneficial. This work is extremely demanding and difficult, and the issues that it raises are complex and hard to resolve. People with dementia deserve the best services and the most skilled therapists. What little they receive generally falls below these standards.

ASSESSMENT FOR PSYCHOTHERAPY

Psychotherapy is not for everyone, even amongst those without a cognitive disability. Therefore, while good listening skills – the basis of psychotherapy – should be a fundamental part of good dementia care in general, we do not believe that all people with a dementing illness should be offered psychotherapy. Before a definite decision is made to offer psychotherapy, then, it is important to make a thorough assessment of the person's ability to benefit from this work. How this assessment is carried out depends in part upon the type of psychotherapy (and there are many forms) that will be used, but despite the differences between different therapists' approaches to assessment, nevertheless some common themes emerge.

Cognitive competence and decline. Two opposing stances concerning the possibility of therapy during the course of dementia have been taken. Some therapists have assumed that interventions such as cognitive therapy that place a premium on verbal skills may be most suited for Alzheimer's disease patients who are more cognitively intact and for those patients in early and mid-dementia who have a degree of self-awareness and insight (e.g. Solomon and Szwabo 1992; Miller 1989). On this basis, where the dementia sufferer is in a more advanced stage of the disease and where the cognitive losses have caused a more significant loss in pleasurable events, then behavioural approaches may be more suitable (Teri and Gallagher-Thompson 1991).

Other therapists have argued that the psychoanalytical defence mechanisms of denial and repression, which serve to protect dementia sufferers from the emotional implications of their illness, result in lack of insight (Cotrell and Lein 1993; Verhey *et al.* 1993). Lack of awareness can thus be taken as an indication of poor dementia care (Kitwood 1990b) and, potentially, the target for a psychotherapeutic intervention.

However, if one of the goals of psychotherapy is to increase levels of insight, then it is possible that for some particularly susceptible individuals this may lead to increased depression. Not only may increases in insight lead, at least initially, to an intensification of emotional reactions, but, without support from the other important people in their life, the dementia sufferer is unlikely to be able to maintain any progress that has been made. Indeed, as we argued in Chapter 8, it may be that for many dementia sufferers denial is the only possible response to the losses that they have experienced and to those which are yet to come.

Personality. As the dementing process is superimposed upon the individual's existing personality it is important to understand their life history and how they have coped with previous crises. Where the person has tended to block out difficulties or pretend that they were not happening, it will be harder for them to begin to address the losses involved in dementia, even with therapeutic help.

What we are saying is 1) all people with dementia should be considered for therapy; although 2) not all, after assessment, will be found able or likely to benefit from it; and 3) even among those who are so able, we must consider the level of environmental support and understanding before therapy is offered and embarked upon.

DIFFERENCES BETWEEN WORKING WITH PEOPLE WITH DEMENTIA AND WITH OTHER PEOPLE

A range of adaptations to therapy have been advocated to cope with the cognitive and verbal deficits of this client group. These include shorter but more frequent sessions and providing patients with either a summary or an audiotape of sessions. In addition, however, it is important to be aware of a range of other changes that may need to be made.

Accommodating verbal deficits. Conversation with dementia sufferers can often lapse into silence as the person with dementia struggles to express him-

or herself. At these points the therapist needs to act almost as a memory bank for clients, reflecting comments back, recalling earlier answers and prompting them to make links (Peach and Duff 1991; Sinason 1992; Yale 1995).

The therapeutic context. Therapists may need to be flexible about where they work so that psychotherapy can occur within a less formal context than usual, for instance while going for a walk or over a cup of tea. Where psychotherapeutic work is taking place in an institution then facilities for confidential interviewing may be difficult to find. It may be necessary to use the patient's room, a staff room or any setting where the patient feels 'safe'.

Therapeutic tensions. Therapists need to be aware of certain tensions that may arise within their work. For instance, psychiatrists, social workers and psychologists are all part of a system that has the potential to deprive dementia sufferers of their liberty and independence. Attempting to act both as someone who may be perceived as a jailer and as confidante can create dangerous tensions within a relationship.

For this reason, the therapist will need to 1) spell out the powers they have or might use that relate to the person's freedom and well-being; 2) negotiate the basis on which they are seeing the person with 3) the person agreeing to be seen and 4) this agreement being reiterated at the start of each session.

There are basically two different forms of psychotherapy: exploratory psychotherapy (where the therapist takes a neutral stance, providing time for the patient to make sense out of what is happening, but without offering advice); and directive therapy (where the therapist attempts to guide or direct the patient according to their sense of what is wrong).

EXPLORATORY THERAPY

The central issues in exploratory psychotherapy concern the therapist's ability to help their client to explore what is happening to them and for them to reach their own understanding. The therapist does not try to impose their own understanding on the client. Both psychodynamic psychotherapy and humanistic therapy (see our description of Resolution Therapy in Chapter 13) can be thought of as exploratory therapies, although there are also significant differences between them.

In considering the use of exploratory therapies with people with dementia we need to be aware of the powerful emotional forces that can be released in this form of work, and of how these emotional forces can be managed successfully.

Containment. Having to confront the personal realities of having dementia creates almost unbearably strong emotional forces. If these are to emerge, then they can only do so within a secure environment in which the therapist is seen to be able to cope with the exploration of these themes. The person with dementia needs to be emotionally held – to be comforted and reassured on an emotional level that their feelings are bearable and that they can be tolerated. This is what analysts call 'containment'. Even though the person with dementia may experience difficulties in consciously remembering their therapist, simply being there on a consistent basis and bearing witness to the person's sense of loss and threat may, in itself, be a steadying intervention.

Coping with the pain of working with dementia sufferers. Because dementia compromises so much of what makes us unique as human beings, working with clients who have dementia can also elicit deep emotional reactions amongst therapists and carers. This is true of whatever form of therapy is used, but for exploratory therapists, the ability to be aware of one's own emotional reaction is vitally important.

Exploratory psychotherapy requires the therapist to react to the dementia sufferer on an empathic basis, and to be aware of the horror of continued neurological decline. We may react to the awfulness of the lives of the people that we work with and to the pain that we too may feel in different ways; some of these are likely to be constructive whilst others may be quite destructive. For instance, some mental health workers may infantilise their patients, acting as if they were small children who needed to be protected from the slightest hurt; alternatively, they may place patients in the position of their own parents, acting out their own ambivalent feelings towards them.

In listening to what people with dementia tell us about themselves we have to listen to the poetical, metaphorical aspects of their language. But this is hard. The emotional pain that can be generated within this form of work can be immense. We need to remember that it is not just the pain of the person with dementia that we are listening to, and it is not just their losses that they are speaking of. These are also our own potential losses, our own future pain. We are listening to people talking about a pain that may well one day be our own or that of our husbands, wives, fathers or mothers. We cannot make this future 'better' in the sense of taking this pain away. We can only try to listen and help the person feel that they have been heard. This is as hard as it is necessary (Sutton and Cheston 1997).

Supporting the grieving process. Any exploratory psychotherapeutic approach to the care of people with dementia needs to provide conditions in which the dementia sufferer can grieve for their losses and be helped to accept the pain of these losses. While it is important not to force someone into confronting issues that they do not feel ready to deal with, at the same time we also need to be able to tolerate extremes of anger and despair. If we, the carers of the people with dementia, cannot bear their sadness and unhappiness then we can hardly expect them to do so.

Working with people in denial. One of the hardest aspects of working with dementia sufferers is trying to work with someone who denies having any form of problem or difficulty despite all the evidence to the contrary. In Part Two of this book we argued that denial is a strategy that people use when threatened by an apparently overwhelming loss. Consequently, rather than seeing denial as part and parcel of the neurological impact of dementia we should view it as a strategy that is both functional and variable.

Thus, denial is often more of a problem for carers and service providers than for the person with dementia. The place that we, as therapists and carers, need to start from is *not* the reality of growing incompetence, bereavement, the loss of skills and so on that we might see. Rather, our starting point must be the reality as experienced by the individual that we are working with. Our task as therapists and carers is to help the person that we are working with 'let go' of the old reality that they are clinging on to, and we can begin to do this by empathising with their fear, terror and despair as they contemplate the real world around them.

Along with the need to begin by empathising with the person with dementia's emotional need to block out the world around them, we also must keep in mind the fact that the use of denial may well place the person that we are working with in physical danger. We cannot simply act as if their imagined world really was the world, as often the person's use of denial means that they do not use services which they and those around them need to use. While it may be emotionally safe to be in a state of denial, being in such a state may also place the person in a physically unsafe environment. Therefore, we have to be honest, own our own reality and where necessary present that reality to our client. Many of these issues are addressed through the case example of Hattie.

Hattie – moving on from denial

In order to illustrate some of these issues we will describe work with Hattie, a woman that one of us (RC) worked with. Hattie was an eighty-three-year-old woman who was admitted to an in-patient ward with an initial diagnosis of Korsakoff's syndrome (dementia related to alcohol abuse – *see* Chapter 2), although this was later changed to a diagnosis of dementia of the Alzheimer's type.

Hattie had been living on her own since the death of her husband three years before. However, recently she had fallen several times, and the last year had seen such a rapid deterioration in her ability to cope for herself that she was admitted for assessment. It quickly became clear that Hattie would be unable to continue to care for herself at home. However, as she was clearly upset by her move to the ward she was referred to a therapy group that RC was establishing with a staff nurse on the ward (Helen Davis).

Hattie angrily maintained that there was nothing wrong with her and that she was only there because the staff did not have enough patients to fill their beds. She regularly announced her intention to go home, and had, on several occasions, found her way out of the ward and tried unsuccessfully to find her way home. The nursing staff who knew Hattie felt that she had very little insight into her own behaviour and mental state.

When Hattie first joined the group she found it hard to sit and listen to other people talking. She seemed to be unhappy when members of the group spoke of difficulties or sadness in their lives. On these occasions she often changed the conversation or interrupted them, saying 'yes, but you've just got to get on with life … the past is past, so there's nothing to be done about it'.

By the sixth session of the group, the group leaders felt that the group as a whole was not addressing the important issues that existed for its members. Within supervision we realised that this was partly because of Hattie's behaviour in the group, but also that it reflected our own discomfort at working within such a restrictive system. This meant that the group had so far failed to address some of the central emotional issues, including Hattie's anger at being on the ward and her wish to leave.

In the next session the group leaders acknowledged to the group that they were part of this wider system. Both Hattie and another group member were able to speak for the first time of their feelings of being prisoners on the ward and of having lost control of their own lives.

continued

The group as a whole became animated in a way that had not been possible before, sharing their common sense of being imprisoned and the strength that they derived from each other's support.

Later, after the group had ended, in an individual session with RC, Hattie commented once again that 'I feel my life's not my own, that I'm a prisoner here. Someone else is living my life'. However, she was able to go on to say that her daughter had taken her to Ocean View residential home and to one other residential home. Hattie remembered that she had liked Ocean View and had decided against the other residential home because they would not let her have her cat there.

For Hattie, it was important to be able to describe the move as being her choice, as this showed that she was still in command of her life and that her independence was not compromised. Perhaps because of this, Hattie was now also able to acknowledge that her own house would be sold and that she would never return there.

In order to help Hattie to adapt to this change in her life a psychology assistant (Susan Byatt) began to work with her on a one-to-one basis. The initial emphasis in this work was on helping Hattie to think back over her life, tell her own life story and grieve for these changes.

Helping Hattie to grieve

There were a number of ways in which we tried to help Hattie to grieve. Much of this process was concerned with her wish to return home:

1. *Giving Hattie as much control over her life as possible.* Hattie often talked about home as if she still lived there, said that she wanted to go home and tried to leave the ward to do so. While her frequent requests to go home were entirely legitimate they needed to be balanced against the fact that the house was up for sale and the competing demands on nursing time. Consequently Susan arranged to take Hattie back to her home at regular points, and also took her to visit a sick relative who had been admitted to hospital.

2. *Expressing her distress.* When Hattie spoke about 'going home' this seemed to be as much about her need to find somewhere that was safe and secure as it was for a real place. Hattie's requests to go home, then, were also signs of her emotional distress. At times the ward staff tried to hide her coat hoping that if she did not see it then she would not be reminded of her wish to leave.

continued

However, as part of Hattie's wish to return home reflected her need to find a more emotionally secure place, taking her coat away actually increased her anxieties and made her more desperate to leave.

3. *Emotional ambivalence.* Hattie's feelings about 'home' were complex. The visits home showed that Hattie was highly ambivalent about returning, at times insisting that she be taken and then changing her mind once arrangements had been made, telling Susan that she was afraid that things would have changed. 'Home', then, represented much more than the stone and mortar of her last address: she told Susan that being at home was about the people there, not the place itself, and often spoke as if she was still living in Newcastle, where she had been brought up, and as if her husband and parents were still alive. This seemed to reflect an inner uncertainty – and the actions surrounding her visits home seemed to be examples of attachment-seeking behaviour (Miesen 1992; 1993).

4. *Acknowledging these feelings.* By talking through these feelings with Susan Hattie was able to move on from her ruminations about leaving the ward and allow herself to be distracted. It was not that these concerns then disappeared completely, because, of course, there was the underlying cognitive deficit to deal with, which meant that before long Hattie would return to these issues and once again demand to go home. But slowly Hattie began to change.

Psychotherapeutic change

Hattie's view of the world changed during her stay on the ward. During her first weeks and months Hattie had been extremely angry about what had happened to her and felt that she was being kept prisoner against her will. She insisted that she would return home and denied that there was any need for her to enter a residential home. Hattie felt, quite realistically, that someone else was making all the decisions about her life and that nobody was telling her what was going to happen to her. Hattie's view of herself was that she did not in any way have any problems that any other elderly person did not experience.

The changes in Hattie's account of herself that occurred were subtle yet quite significant. Hattie came to recognise that her house had been sold and that she was going to live in Ocean View. She moved from demanding to go home permanently to asking to visit her house, acknowledging that it had been sold.

continued

Hattie's psychological state was, however, extremely varied, and there were times when it appeared that nothing had moved forward. In many ways this was to be expected – anyone who, like Hattie, is grieving the loss of so many precious things will have times when, emotionally, they feel themselves to be back at square one. Hattie's grieving was complicated by her severe memory loss – she found it hard to hold on to the facts about her life. Consequently, she was much more reactive to these inevitable emotional swings than would otherwise be the case, and it was much harder for her to remind herself about what had really happened.

For Hattie, then, denial and protest were gradually replaced by emotional despair and pain. This lead her to confabulate – to fill in the gaps in her emotional world by recalling to life past places in which she felt secure and past people who gave her hope. When she talked about her husband and parents as if they were still alive, this seemed to arise from a process of wish fulfilment, filling the emotional emptiness within her. At the same time there were many moments of reality and of longing for a brighter future at Ocean View.

The final stages of this process – of resolution and reinvesting her emotional energies in a new future – were not possible for Hattie until she left the ward. During her stay Hattie resolutely refused to accept the ward as her home. She refused, for instance, to take in pictures of her family, as she did not want to accept the ward as a home, however temporary. Six months after her move to Ocean View she seemed to be much more settled than she had ever been on the ward – she rarely asked to go home and seemed to be pleased with her new life with her cat.

Resolving conflicts from the past. Validation Therapy (VT) is still probably the most widely known form of psychotherapy with dementia sufferers. These ideas have been put forward by Naomi Feil (1990, 1992, 1993) and are based on the assumption that disoriented elderly people return to the past in an attempt to resolve unfinished conflicts by expressing feelings that have previously been hidden. Feil suggests that the enormity of the losses associated with dementia may well affect the dementia sufferer's most profound relationships. Consequently, the goal of the Validation therapist is to validate what is said by acknowledging the emotion that lies behind the words and then bringing out the emotional conflict underlying the apparently confused behaviour.

VT, then, involves accepting the reality as it is experienced by that person and empathising with that experience. The therapist is said to need to enter imaginatively into the feelings and perceptions of the disoriented person and focus on the emotional rather than the factual content of what people say.

Feil's ideas have been the subject of some criticism (e.g. Stokes and Goudie 1990; Morton 1997). In Feil's later writings there is a strong sense that disorientation is synonymous with dementia and that it arises, in part, from the failure of the individual to resolve previous life stages. In this book we have preferred to emphasise that the emotional torture that many dementia sufferers undoubtedly experience arises from their experiences of dementia.

DIRECTIVE PSYCHOTHERAPY

The most common form of directive psychotherapy is Cognitive and Behavioural Therapy (CBT) (Beck 1976). These ideas have been used with dementia sufferers to pursue a number of therapeutic goals:

Altering dysfunctional thoughts. Teri and Gallagher-Thompson (1991) described how, over an average of 16 to 20 sessions, patients were encouraged to identify and then to challenge their cognitive errors, generating more adaptive ways of viewing specific situations and events. Although it takes some time for patients with dementia to master these skills, in time they were said to have done so and to have found them useful.

Increasing positive reinforcement and reducing negative reinforcement. Teri and Gallagher-Thompson also suggested that depression is maintained by a lack of positive experiences and an excess of aversive experiences. Accordingly, the aim of their interventions is to redress the balance. After the behavioural rationale is explained to both the clients and their relatives, realistic and explicit goals are established. Behavioural change principles are then taught to the relative and, as far as possible, to the client.

Achieving a sense of control and agency. Several authors have argued that it may be therapeutic to help people with dementia regain some degree of mastery of the environment by helping them problem-solve and communicate their decisions to their family.

Increasing coping skills. LaBarge and Trtanj (1995) described a group intervention in which clients developed both practical coping skills (such as asking for help and using simple mnemonics) and intrapsychic coping skills (most importantly, a greater sense of self-efficacy and the use of humour).

Stress management

A variety of interventions aimed at reducing symptoms of anxiety have been proposed. These include teaching relaxation techniques, using simple meditation exercises, and cognitive training using visual imagery (Haggerty 1990). Welden and Yesavage (1982), for instance, found that relaxation training reduced anxiety and improved the memory of elderly patients with dementia, including some with Alzheimer's disease.

Social constructionist approaches to identity

While psychodynamic approaches to identity focus on internal structures and the patient's relationship with significant people, the social constructionist approach that we outlined earlier in this book views identity as something that is achieved through social interaction. There has, indeed, been an increasing amount of work looking at the ways in which a sense of social and personal identity can be maintained by dementia sufferers (e.g. Buchanan and Middleton 1993, 1994, 1996; Cheston 1996; Sabat and Harré 1992).

One of the starting places for a social constructionist approach to dementia has been the examination of what we mean by 'memory'. We described, in earlier chapters, how the standard psychological ways of conceptualising the process of remembering in terms of the reliability of a person's memory have prevented us from asking important questions about the *process* of remembering. Instead of being concerned with 'truthfulness' we should be more concerned with finding out what a person achieves by talking about the past in the way that they do.

A central tenet of discursive or social constructionist approaches is that the process of remembering has to be seen in the context in which it takes place – with what remembering allows us to do. One of the things that having a memory allows us to do is construct a narrative that helps us to make sense of our life and communicate with others.

So, for instance, the two of us who are writing this book meet regularly to discuss progress. At these meetings we recall from our previous discussions what it is that we want to write in this book and why we want to write it (even though our separate memories are quite distinct, and will change, grow and shrink over time). As we talk about past meetings and past agreements and experiences, so each of us tries to persuade the other that some things should be left in and others taken out. It is through such talk about the past that people are able to move others towards accepting their versions of events or create a shared sense of belonging. Talking about the past, future and present enables us to become and remain social beings.

Let us apply this line of reasoning now to people with dementia. One of us has been involved in research describing how individuals with dementia are able to both talk about the past as a way of making sense of their present experiences and comment upon this process (Cheston 1996). Two of the people with dementia that this research focuses upon describe recreating the past through talk as an active coping strategy to overcome feelings of being useless and as a way of making sense of the world. Similarly, Buchanan and Middleton (1994) have examined how within a reminiscence group talk about the past, and in particular talk about occasions on which participants have been able to help other people, achieves a number of functions. Participants use such talk, for instance, to establish a shared sense of social identity and as a means of establishing their entitlement to care.

A fundamental part of good dementia care, then, involves allowing people with dementia to have the time and the space not just to reminisce or talk about their common past with others, but to talk about their own lives. Sharing these memories with others in the context of a group is of great value – something that has long been recognised by those using Reminiscence Therapy. In this way of working dementia sufferers are prompted to recall memories, often through the use of aids such as collections of photographs of the local area. Social constructionist ideas, however, suggest that this should be allied to the process of creating a shared conception of 'who we are'. For instance, Moyes and Christie (1998a) have described how the men at the Gala Day Hospital (see Chapter 13) formed a group in which they talked about themselves as 'the Gala Boys' – a group of men who in their youth had fought together for King and country and had similar experiences.

Reminiscence about the past, then, needs to be viewed as a way of forming a social identity. Reminiscence or storytelling is a social act – it is something that takes place in front of an audience. Telling a story can provide a shared sense of social identity and can be a means of providing a therapeutic continuity to individuals' lives. In the stories that people with dementia tell about the past we can see echoes of the losses they have suffered. For instance, at the beginning of a group for people with dementia run by Laura Sutton, a clinical psychologist working in Southampton, the stories that were told reflected themes of uncertainty and struggle, many being set in the Second World War and using metaphors of the participants being 'in the wars again' and unsure about the 'officers'' ability. As the group progressed through the twelve weekly meetings, however, the stories that the participants told began to change. They began to talk of how the camaraderie that they all felt had got them through such difficult times, of how the officers had done more than they thought, and, talking of the battle, of the time when they were waiting to 'go over the top' (Sutton and Cheston 1997).

Using a collage to develop a life story

Storytelling has a vitally important role to play in enabling individuals to preserve a sense of who they are. Life-story work is a formalised way of taking people with dementia through their own life story. These stories can be bound together to form a book, recorded on tape and illustrated with photographs and other visual prompts (Jarvis 1997).

Karen Jarvis, a Community Psychiatric Nurse working for Hull and Holderness Community Health Trust, has described how she used collages in her work with one of her clients, Mr Greaney, whose wife had died recently during a period of respite care. Following her death, Mr Greaney, who had a history of alcohol abuse, began to drink heavily and became suicidal.

Karen visited weekly to develop a therapeutic relationship and allow Mr Greaney to express his feelings about his situation and explore his bereavement. Over a period of several months Mr Greaney began to tell 'his story', which mainly concerned his experiences during his career at sea, and the war. His body language on these occasions changed from a slumped, seemingly uninterested posture to one in which he became animated. On one occasion he recalled a sea voyage of which he obviously felt proud to have been part. The voyage had involved the collection of wild animals from Africa and their subsequent delivery as the first ever consignment for Bristol Zoo. He was visibly excited, upright and pacing about the room while he described the animals and the arrival at Bristol docks in 1946. Karen felt that Mr Greaney was tapping into his old self, the person he had once been.

Through the course of Mr Greaney's therapy Karen made attempts to develop the narrative still further. This seemed to require something more tangible and in an adaptation of the more usual verbal life review work she began to create a collage with Mr Greaney.

continued

Collage is the art of gathering images from a variety of sources and pasting them down onto a flat surface to make a single creative work. Some people begin a collage with a set theme or concept, then select images that best express it. Titles are particularly important to this method because they provide a concise synopsis of the collage's significance.

Once the images are selected they are pasted down, as either an original piece or a photocopy from an original. Images are cut to fit together as in a jigsaw puzzle.

Karen discussed this idea with Mr Greaney and he was keen that other people might see him as he was in his prime, in the career he enjoyed so much. They decided to create a collage representing his life experiences. He selected photographs and other documentation which he wanted to include and Karen was able to find other relevant illustrative material which depicted his stories. Mr Greaney wanted all of the material, including the photographs, to be slightly smaller than the main document – his passport. This seemed to firmly stamp his identity on the collage, becoming its dominant feature.

The process of completing this work seemed to enable Mr Greaney to manage his grief and separation anxiety. He was more able to function independently, cooking for himself and seeing friends again. From having a history of alcohol abuse, he stopped drinking completely.

Although Mr Greaney did not have dementia, exactly the same visual way of working has also been successful with clients who do suffer from dementia, whose short-term memory is very poor but whose long-term memory is good. Having a pictorial reference to the times in their life that they can remember has shown beneficial effects in mood and allows clients to reaffirm their identities. Negotiation with the client seems to be the key to producing a successful piece of work. It is important to allow the client to remain the sole editor of their work. There is also the added bonus that these life stories can be of great interest to relatives and friends who may not otherwise have known of the stories behind the pictures.

In Chapter 9 we described the concept of positioning – the idea that each of us uses social interactions to present ourselves as being a particular sort of person. However, the sorts of relationships available to many people with dementia, especially those in residential or nursing care, rarely allow them to position themselves in ways that enable them to feel valued or needed. As we noted in the last section, forms of care should actively encourage such opportunities, helping people with dementia to continue previous relationships (for instance as a marital and sexual partner, a parent and grandparent, or a friend and confidant) and establish new relationships. We could try, therefore, to provide opportunities for people with dementia to be oral historians or teachers, providing local schools with accounts of the last war, the depression and so on – which places them in the position of valued informants on society.

Structuring care to maintain personhood

There is a strong conceptual and practical overlap between the social constructionist approach to dementia care and that put forward by Tom Kitwood. His writings focus on how dementia care practices can act to either strengthen or undermine an individual's sense of personhood. Good dementia care aims to buttress dementia sufferers' sense of themselves as people of worth and value, and may thus be inherently psychotherapeutic (Kitwood 1990b).

In his influential book, *Dementia Reconsidered* (1997), Tom Kitwood set out ten ways in which forms of care could be organised to enable a dementia sufferer's personhood to be strengthened:

- *recognition* – the person who has dementia is recognised and affirmed as a unique person.
- *negotiation* – the person who has dementia is consulted about their preferences, desires and needs.
- *collaboration* – two or more people share a common task, working together to achieve a common aim.
- *play* – the exercise of spontaneity and self-expression, an experience that has value in itself.
- *timalation* – in creating this word, Tom Kitwood was trying to capture a form of interaction in which the prime modality is sensuous or sensual, for example aromatherapy or massage.
- *celebration* – this refers not simply to special occasions but to any moment at which life is experienced as especially joyful.
- *relaxation* – this may require social and even physical contact, although for some people with dementia it may be possible to relax in solitude.
- *validation* – Tom Kitwood used this word in a similar way to Naomi Feil, that is to say, to refer to the use of a high degree of empathy to

understand a person's entire frame of reference, even if this is chaotic, paranoid or filled with delusions.

- *holding* – this refers to the 'holding' of emotions. In a psychological sense, to 'hold' means to provide a 'container' in which hidden traumas can be revealed and extreme vulnerability exposed in the confidence that the emotions associated with this will be respected and not rejected.

- *facilitation* – to enable the person to do what he or she wants to do but cannot. This requires empathy to sense both what the person desires and also just what he or she cannot manage, without imposing more.

In addition, Kitwood outlined two other patterns of personhood-sustaining interaction, both of which originate from the person with dementia rather than their carer:

- *creation* – here the person with dementia offers something to the social setting spontaneously, for instance by singing or dancing.

- *giving* – this refers to the person with dementia expressing concern or appreciation.

An example of giving was the Gift group run at Riverview centre (Age Concern), Plymouth, in the winters of 1996 and 1998 with the aim of 'reversing the gift relationship' (Titmuss 1997). This has two operating principles. First, in any chronic sickness, all the giving – of presents, time and energy – is from relatives and friends of the sick person. Therefore, if the sick person can create a present of real quality (not a present which requires the apology of being sick) this will be a powerful statement of agency and giving. Second, even a person with severe dementia can make a sophisticated, high-quality present as long as the creation of that present is sufficiently broken down into small steps. With the support of the centre head, Denise Gregson, these aims were very successfully achieved on both occasions with two groups of six clients with moderate or severe dementia. The first group was led by the deputy head, Yvonne Todson, and assistant psychologists Judith Horrocks and Tracey Bullock, and the second by three staff, Pat Holden, Patrick Baker and a student, Ann Parsons, backed up by Emma Snelling, assistant psychologist. Each member of the group chose one person for whom to make a present and wrote some Christmas cards. The biggest problem was ensuring that the presents got delivered, so a party was held to which the recipients of the presents were invited. They were given their wrapped presents with strict instructions not to open them until Christmas.

The power of reversing the gift relationship was shown by the tears in the eyes of some of the relatives as the clients gave them their gifts. For one relative, the gift became particularly treasured – her mother died soon after and so the present was the last she ever received from her.

Establishing identity without words

As the person's ability to describe and control their environment through the use of words decreases, so the importance of the environment itself in determining their behaviour increases (Lawton 1980a and b). This is a key point to grasp with services to people with dementia. Increasingly, if you like, the staff have to provide and create the quality in their client's lives.

Bender and Bauckham (1998) and Bender, Bauckham and Norris (1999) provide a framework for moving away from the verbal (see Table 14.1).

Table 14.1 Getting through to a person when you are not able to use verbal means of communication	
Medium or modality	*Examples*
Visual representation	Photographs, slides
Smell/taste	Smell kits Types of food
Visual direct	Looking at objects of autobiographical meaning Painting pictures
Music	Familiar tunes, records from times past Making music
Tactile	Touching physical objects Manipulating materials to get sensory experiences, e.g. planting bulbs, making cakes Feeling various textures Painting Massage

In terms of maintaining identity, reminiscence work is important, as it allows access to past identity and, hopefully, some continuity. Bender, Bauckham and Norris (1999) provide many examples of how reminiscence work can be modified to become less verbal and more tactile and auditory. Other ideas for this middle range of difficulties are to be found in Stokes and Goudie (1990).

One way of relating reminiscence to identity is a 'Getting to know you' group in which reminiscence is used to encourage the person to present and develop their identity. Its rationale came from attempts to develop Erikson's (1977) ideas of psychosocial stages and tasks for use in a group format (Bender 1997a; Bender, Bauckham and Norris 1999). We found the concepts of autonomy, trust, industry etc. quite hard for the clients we were working with to understand. A 10-session group based on chronological chunks – early years, going to school, first job, leisure and courtship etc. – is far more accessible and far more appropriate for people who have dementia.

The concept is also easily understood by staff. Supervision and clinical follow-up resources need to be available, as traumatic events are described. It is an excellent way for keyworkers to gain a much deeper understanding of their clients. This kind of group, suitably paced by experienced group workers, can be used as long as the members have some speech, even where the cognitive damage is extensive.

When individuals are in the more advanced stages of dementia and verbal behaviour is limited, then communication through physical means such as holding, stroking and touching may also help to provide a primitive sense of comfort (Feil 1993). At these points, just being there and responding in a sensitive and comforting way, as a parent comforts their child by gently rocking and stroking, may meet a very primitive need to be comforted and have one's distress acknowledged. We will return to this theme shortly.

Lessening information-processing problems

We suggested in Chapter 12 that conventional assessments often confuse a person's dislocation from their social world with a reduction in their cognitive capacity, with the result that the person being assessed is likely to be seen as having a poorer memory than is actually the case. We can extend this argument to consider the effects of being in a nursing home or in-patient ward upon dementia sufferers. All too often these environments insulate the people within them from the external world. They are, in effect, small institutions which impose their own tempo upon the small world within them: for example, staff rotas, meetings and ward rounds and the pattern of getting up, getting dressed, having breakfast and so on. This pattern is almost entirely independent of what is happening outside the ward or home.

All of our memories are, at least in part, held within social events. The Remembrance Service on 11 November is one example of this – a socially organised act of remembering. Memories are, therefore, socially maintained – and without our social memory we lose something of our social identity. All of us learn to orientate towards temporal markers within our worlds – and if this is the world of work, then the pattern of events in work is matched by a pattern of events outside work. But this is not true for dementia sufferers who are in-patients on wards or who live in other institutions. Their pattern of life is almost entirely shaped by the ward or hospital in which they live.

What is needed, then, are methods of orienting dementia sufferers to the social patterns of events around them. This is more than Reality Orientation – it recognises the social nature of memory and of remembering, rather than being concerned to orientate people to the reality around them. For instance, work by Backman (1992) showed that making days memorable increased the ease with which events were remembered. Similarly, Mills (1997) has suggested that when events have a personal relevance they are more easily remembered.

Bender, Bauckham and Norris (1999) have described one way of working that draws upon these ideas. Unison groups (Bender 1995) are an attempt to link the person to the seasons and the calendar. They aim to use basic changes – from summer to winter – and strongly emotive occasions – Armistice Day, Christmas Day and so on – to access the memories of people with severe dementia and engage them in work (Bender and Bauckham 1998). The process of remembering these important social events within the context of a group of one's peers creates a shared sense of purpose and identity. This is facilitated by the group leaders who encourage creativity and communication between members.

The importance of using all our senses

So far we have concentrated on helping individuals to retain a sense of who they are through the use of language. For dementia sufferers, however, the ability to use language deteriorates gradually. At this point it is important to turn to other forms of working and use other forms of stimulation. The Sensory Stimulation groups that Bender, Bauckham and Norris (1999) described utilised a wide variety of materials that were pleasant to touch and feel. Mowle-Clarke, Bender and Brown (1992) – a physiotherapist, psychologist and occupational therapist respectively – ran two twelve-session 'feelie-wheel' groups where two groups – of women and men working independently, as they came from segregated wards – each made half of the wheel, using a great number of different materials. Interestingly, pleasantness of touch and feel did nothing for the men who needed materials such as wood and iron – elements from their working life – to stimulate and engage them.

Larissa Kempenaar, a physiotherapist, and Christine McNamara, a research nurse at Ailsa Hospital, Ayrshire, assessed their patients according to which sense was still most acute and most likely to respond to stimulation (smell and taste; hearing; vision). They gave regular weekly sessions, of an average of 45 minutes' duration, using that modality, and then taught the person's carer to do so. They are in the process of researching the benefits of this approach.

Using Taste and Smell

Mrs W has a severe cognitive impairment and attends a day hospital. Her behaviour is challenging, as she is disruptive within group situations. She is dysphasic and constantly mutters a stream of what seem to be nonsensical words. She can be very demanding of staff attention and hits out at staff and fellow patients when this is not given. She lives with her daughter, who also finds her behaviour difficult to manage at times.

Mrs W had been given various types of individual sensory stimulation. During these sessions Mrs W was unable to settle and at times became physically aggressive towards the therapist. Finally a smell and taste session was tried. This turned out to be her 'preferred sense'. She was able to participate in the tasting of various foodstuffs for a period of about 45 minutes. During this time staff offered her small amounts of a variety of foodstuffs on a teaspoon, allowing her time to respond verbally or non-verbally. She appeared to enjoy this, smiling when she tasted something she liked and grimacing when she did not. Staff in the ward noticed that during the time of the programme Mrs W appeared less agitated than usual, she was remarkably less agitated on the way home in the ambulance. Mrs W's daughter felt that her mother was more alert. Mrs W had reinstated her habit of helping to set the tea dishes and wash them, something that Mrs W had stopped doing the previous year. (Kempenaar and McNamara 1998, p.29)

Summary of main points

- Dementia is a process that undermines a sufferer's ability to preserve a sense of themselves as a unique and valuable being. In this chapter we have outlined three different ways – the psychodynamic, the social constructionist and personhood – of thinking about identity or the self. Each one of these viewpoints emphasises the importance of the social world that individuals live within. Consequently, it is important that patterns of dementia care allow people with dementia the opportunity to create and to maintain their own identity.
- As the person's skills and verbal abilities decrease, so the importance of the environment in determining the quality of the person's life increases.
- Identity work needs to move away from exclusively verbal methods to incorporate methods using other means of communication such as sound and music.
- However, the need to try to reach the other through words and conversation, wherever possible, remains.
- Identity work is certainly easier when the person can use symbols and words, but the need for such work remains just as great when they cannot.

CHAPTER 15

Changing Systems
of Service Delivery

In this chapter we examine the implications of the person-focused approach
for the organisation and delivery of services to people with dementia. First of
all we focus on the place where the majority of people with dementia are to
be found: in their homes in the community. In the second part of the chapter
we move on to look at institutional settings – the day centre or day hospital,
the residential home and the nursing home.

We look at the requirements for good institutional care – training,
changing the environmental atmosphere and methods of ongoing evaluation
that involve the client – and review some possible improvements. We end the
chapter with a short checklist of points regarding good practice concerning
the client and the maintenance of their relationships.

Services to people living with dementia in the community

Often, books about people with dementia focus almost exclusively on institutional settings and, in doing so, forget that the majority of people with
dementia live in their own homes. Gordon and Spicker (1997), for instance,
in a survey of the Tayside area of Scotland (1992–1994), found that 56 per
cent of people with dementia were living in the community. Similarly,
Kavanagh *et al.* (1993) reported a figure for the whole of England in
1985/1986 of 63 per cent living in their own homes.

The first place in which we need to organise services, then, is in the
community. As we have argued throughout this book, these services need:

- to focus on the person with dementia
- to be readily available on a long-term basis.

Organising services in this way would change considerably the framework within which the services are currently delivered. This is, however, the only real way in which the various parts of the family system can be supported and the needs of the person with dementia can begin to be met.

Making services readily available to all people with dementia living in the community

One of the most noteworthy findings of a series of community surveys is the large number of people who have dementia and who live on their own without an informal carer.

> There is little agreement between studies on the proportion of people with dementia in the community without an informal carer: 5 percent (Badger, Cameron and Evers, 1990) 18 percent (McCullough, 1980) 20–26 percent (Levin, Sinclair and Gorbach, 1983, 1989) and 34 percent (Wenger, 1994). In Tayside, we found that around one in five of community residents with dementia apparently lacked an involved informal carer. (Gordon and Spicker 1997, p.45)

Taking the average of these studies suggests that one in five people with dementia look after themselves in the community. Arguably the most effective way to support these people is to increase their general standard of living and ensure that sufficient resources and finances are available to *all* old people in the community. This may seem rather mundane, more an economic task than a psychological one. However, a person's quality of life is to a large extent determined by their standard of living, so we need to channel the necessary resources to all older people, including those with dementia living on their own in their own homes.

We cannot separate, then, the care that people living with dementia in their own homes need from the wider needs of older people in general for a caring society, a decent pension, affordable heating and so on. This is a political and economic decision, even if the arguments compelling us towards it are psychological and clinical ones.

Making services available on a long-term basis

It is clearly important that people who may have dementia are assessed as early as possible so as to rule out alternative, treatable causes of their problems. An early diagnosis also enables a dialogue to start between the person with dementia and their relatives, their GP and other potentially important people in their lives.

If we are to attempt to engage with people with dementia at an early point after their diagnosis and to focus our services on meeting their needs, then one of our aims should be to empower them to manage their lives. The person with dementia should have access to information about their diagnosis and prognosis, and should be able to control who else has access to this information. Rather than adopt a paternalistic approach to their well-being we should see the person with dementia as a responsible agent, and also as someone who, at least in the early stages, is still capable of living with the consequences of their actions. There is a difficult balance to strike between removing responsibility (in the interests of protecting someone who cannot care for themselves) and taking away significant control over their lives (thereby reducing that person to the status of a child). This involves a difficult assessment of the conflicting risks that are involved.

What is clear from the present scene is that the advertising of new drugs is making increasing numbers of people go to their GPs for help with memory difficulties — and these are often people in relationships. Many of these people will *not* be suffering from dementia but from treatable conditions such as depression. For those who are we need to develop ways of working which help them to maintain a sense of themselves as coherent and valuable people. At the same time, the person with dementia may also have to handle considerable anxiety and depression on the part of their relative in addition to their own grief and bewilderment at the loss of their skills.

What is very evident from our clinical work is how 'hot' and dynamic these relationships between people with dementia and their relatives are, and how actively negotiation and re-negotiation are taking place. All of this takes place in the context of a previous relationship, which for many will not have been without tensions and traumas. Inquiring and learning about 'the small print of the marriage contract', to quote a useful phrase of Colin Murray Parkes (Bender 1976), allows us to understand how previous difficulties were tackled and what commitments and attitudes towards illness and support each are bringing into play now.

The person with dementia, then, is living and interacting within a network of complex, ambivalent and highly-charged relationships. Like all of us, the person with dementia is trying actively to make sense of and negotiate these relationships, however limited their ability to do so.

Mrs Smith – living with frustration

Mrs Smith was manifestly at risk in the home that she had lived in for many years with her now deceased husband. To help keep her in the community, which was her wish, her daughter, husband and young child moved in. This seemed a logical step as the house was large.

Mrs Smith, however, did not approve of her daughter's child-rearing, and most of all, deeply resented being looked after and monitored. During counselling sessions she was frequently in tears. Unable to change the situation, she displaced her frustration onto the day hospital staff, which was tolerated; her unhappiness also resulted in wandering and some aggression towards her family, which led eventually to hospitalisation. Placed then in a residential home, she became much calmer and formed a good relationship with the domestic staff, helping, to the best of her ability, with household chores. Once again, she was able to be in a relationship in which her identity needs were respected.

A variety of therapeutic services, then, should be available to both the patient and their relative(s) on their own, and as a family (for a review of family therapy with people with dementia *see* Benbow *et al.* 1993). Similarly, it is important that advocacy be made available to people with dementia, just as it is to people with other mental illnesses (cf. Burton 1997).

If the person with dementia is trying to make sense of difficult relationships and failing then the resultant stress may well precipitate further cognitive decline. If mental health professionals and other agencies are to make a contribution to clarifying relationships such as those of Mrs Smith then support needs to be both readily available and long term. While it is important to maintain the *system* that supports the person with dementia the prime aim of services should be to understand and support the *person* with dementia. The principal client of these services must be the person with dementia. In many cases their needs will be met most easily by supporting their relationship with their relatives, although as we have said, the needs of relatives and people with dementia are not always synonymous.

To summarise our understanding of work with people who are living in the community and have dementia, the services need to be:

- readily available
- long term

- focused on the person with dementia (which considerably changes the framework within which the services are delivered)
- delivered in a way which ensures that the various parts of the family system and the system itself are supported.

Working in institutions with people who have dementia

The structure of services for people who have dementia tends to be top-heavy – weighted towards institutional settings, which are the most labour intensive and thus utilise the most financial and material resources. From the ideas that we have set out so far in this book certain basic principles have emerged:

1. Dementia sufferers need to be seen as active agents. That is to say, they are engaged both in an active struggle to cope with the threat to their identity posed by the direct and the indirect effects of dementia, and also in dealing with the emotional trauma involved in dementia, including the need to grieve for their losses.

2. The active management of identity, if it is to be successful, involves the person assimilating the knowledge that they have dementia into their sense of who they are (their self-concept or identity) without being overwhelmed by the knowledge. The essential elements of who they are remain, and the person and those around them should be able to identify personal continuity.

3. The risk is that this process is not completed successfully and that awareness is either shut out completely or the person is overwhelmed by this awareness and withdraws from the world.

4. The social context within which people who suffer from dementia are cared for needs to be one which encourages dementia sufferers to cope and to manage their illness in as effective a way as they possibly can. In particular, people with dementia need to be seen as capable of both emotional growth and change, and of maintaining a coherent identity into the later stages of the illness.

5. Services for dementia sufferers and their carers, therefore, need to be organised so that they assist in this process. They need to enable the individual to keep their sense of self and also to recognise the deep emotional trauma that is involved.

6. As most services currently stand, there will rarely be enough therapeutically skilled dementia care workers (regardless of their professional labels) to provide the intensive and skilled inputs needed by

each person with dementia. And indeed, to strive for such a goal may be misguided, because, as we discussed in Chapter 2 in the context of dementia, it is the ethos of the environment in which care is delivered that is of the greatest importance in determining the client's quality of care. As well as trying to change the training of individual professionals, then, we need to be able to help those people who work within institutions to change the ethos of their units.

At the risk of repeating ourselves, it is unrealistic to expect meaningful change to occur if we only try to change the way that individuals within systems operate. We need to do more than this and change the way that *systems* work, so that the culture of care within systems such as Social Service departments and the NHS, as well as institutions such as nursing homes and wards, all attend to the emotional and identity needs of dementia sufferers.

Improving the quality of care

We will now go on to examine various ways in which services can begin to improve the quality of the care that they provide. Part of this involves evaluating services from the points of view of the people receiving that care – the people with dementia. We will start by considering ways of improving care through staff training.

Raising awareness of the need for change: staff training and teaching

Identifying the training or teaching needs of staff should start from an appreciation of the needs – especially the unmet needs – of the clients. We have begun to see a significant increase in the quality and number of training packages available. The precise sort of training that is offered will ultimately depend upon the training needs of the staff concerned.

PERSON-CENTRED CARE AND DEMENTIA CARE MAPPING

One of the most well-known forms of staff training is that founded on person-centred care and Dementia Care Mapping (DCM) run either by the Bradford Research Group or by the growing band of trainers who have been licensed by them. These courses emphasise the need to focus on maintaining the personhood of the person with dementia through an awareness of the subtle social dynamics of care. DCM is both a way of raising awareness and of evaluating the quality of care that is being offered (Bradford Dementia Group 1998).

DCM is a system of structured observation in which the mappers sit unobtrusively in a public place within a ward or home. Mappers normally work in a team, with each mapper trying to 'map' the day of perhaps three or four clients. Every five minutes a mapper will record the form of activity that each client has been predominantly engaged in, using an alphabetical code. At the same time he or she records the quality of care received by each individual on a scale from plus five to minus five. Finally, there is also the opportunity for mappers to record examples of any remarks that staff make which might impact negatively upon the personhood of the dementia sufferers with whom they are working. These are known as personal detractions, or PDs.

At the end of the period of mapping, which should have lasted for at least six hours, the mappers add up the different scores and then feed back the results to those members of staff who have been working with the dementia sufferers on that day. One of the great strengths of this way of working is that the mappers should quite quickly be in a position to give relatively detailed feedback to staff about the quality of care that the dementia sufferers have received. DCM is therefore quite a versatile instrument – it can act both as a means of evaluating the quality of care that an institution provides and also as a means of giving very good, accurate feedback to the staff.

AWARENESS OF ATTACHMENT NEEDS

While DCM is undoubtedly the most comprehensive form of training and service evaluation available in the UK today, there are other methods of teaching which attempt to address related issues. One package of teaching that has begun to make an impact is the work of a team at the University of Southampton, which stresses the role of attachment (Mills *et al.* 1998).

The course that they devised was taught in two residential homes for the elderly. It consisted of 18 weekly three-hour sessions over the course of nine months, covering a variety of issues including attachment experiences, communicating with the person with dementia, death and dying, and caring for people who are different in some important respect (e.g. gays, lesbians and those from ethnic minorities). Following this work, the 18-week course was reduced to eight weeks and taught in a third home.

Although there were several written assignments on the course, the major piece of evaluated work was an in-depth case study of one of the residents that the staff worked with. A central feature of these case studies was the attempt that course participants had made to integrate their knowledge of attachment behaviour into their understanding of the individual clients. It was their chance to integrate theory and practice.

The completion of the case studies consolidated changes in care practice that were already being made. Carers reported feeling closer to these people through greater knowledge of their life histories and noted that this aided communication between them. In the third home that the team worked with, alterations were made to the care plans of five of the eight residents included in the case study exercise.

AWARENESS OF DIFFERENCES: GENDER AND DISABILITY

A rather different method of training has been developed by Bender and Horton (1999). Noting that the great majority of workers in the field of dementia are female, they focused on the triad of self, gender and disability. They listed 20 important aspects of the female role – being a daughter, being expected to work, being expected to marry and have children etc.

These roles are discussed in small training groups of four to six students. The students might be care assistants, social work students or Project 2000 nursing students, all women. Each student then interviews one woman aged around 20, one of 40, one of 60 and one with mild to moderate dementia to ascertain their experiences of these aspects of the female role. In this way they realise what women of very different age cohorts have in common; how they differ; how the person with dementia has had similar experiences to the other women; and the extent to which their present position as a person with dementia is affecting them.

Initial results with social work students using this method have been very encouraging, with the students showing a far greater interest in and understanding of dementia at the end of the course than at the beginning. Particularly pleasing was the development of friendships between the students and the clients. The clients also reported that the experience of being interviewed on their experiences and views was rewarding.

COUNSELLING AND LISTENING SKILLS

So far we have looked at training schemes aimed at providing a deeper under-standing of dementia and dementia services. The unit may also need to look at improving the listening and communication skills of the staff. Staff need to understand non-verbal communication, how to communicate emotions, how to listen actively and, we would suggest, basic counselling skills. (Nelson-Jones 1990 and Egan 1994 are useful guides to this area.)

An attempt to train staff in the theory and practice of counselling people with dementia is being undertaken in the Plymouth area in spring 1999 by Gert Landers and Mike Bender as a development of the Companions Club (Bender *et al.* 1999). Gert Landers trains counsellors for CRUSE, the organisation for widows and widowers (Torrie 1970), so some of the new course will use material similar to that used on his training courses. It will be based on the premise, outlined in Chapter 10 of this book, that the central feature of handling dementia is coming to terms with loss. Emphasis will be placed on non-verbal communication and Rogerian concepts such as empathy and unconditional positive regard. The initial teaching time will be 30 hours, spread over ten afternoons, with supervision being essential for those who wish to practise such counselling.

Changing the environment – attending to the context of training

Whatever form of training package is arrived at, it is important to ensure that training occurs within a context that will allow the ideas that are central to the teaching to make an impact on the behaviour of staff:

THE IMPORTANCE OF STAFF SELECTION

Training and support can help staff to develop the skills and awareness necessary for good quality dementia care, but only if they already have some of the qualities that are required for this form of work. The most important abilities are those of empathy, respect for older adults and the ability to value people regardless of any disability. Such attitudes – central therapeutic ingredients, to use Carl Rogers' term (Truax and Carkhuff 1967) – are quite separate from training. What training can do is to help staff to communicate their respect and valuing more effectively and in a more focused manner.

WORKING WITH THE WHOLE SYSTEM

There is little point in training individual members of staff if after this training they return to an old culture of care in which there is very little possibility of change occurring. Change happens most consistently when the whole system is involved in training. For instance, in a ward, it is important to try to involve everyone, from managers and consultants to staff nurses, primary nurses and nursing auxiliaries to kitchen staff and cleaners. When, as a result of such training, changes are agreed upon, then it is important to arrange a time schedule for these to occur and for future dates to review progress.

Evaluation

So training by itself is not enough. For changes to occur, a viewpoint that is independent of staff and management needs to be heard. We need to evaluate these changes from the perspective of those upon whom the changes are supposed to impact most – the people with dementia being cared for.

All services need regular evaluation – or more exactly, all services should be involved in ongoing evaluation. Historically, it has been the voices of the medical profession and other powerful vested interests that have dominated the evaluation of services; consequently, these interests have shaped service provision for people with dementia and their carers. Yet it is important that any service evaluation should focus on the opinions and views of people with dementia. We are not talking about a big research design. Indeed, the most effective and sustainable forms of evaluation occur on a small scale.

Briefly, we can distinguish between those methods which attempt to enable clients with dementia to participate in the evaluation of the services that they receive and those which attempt to evaluate services from the perspective of the dementia sufferer without necessarily sampling their views directly. Research in this area is still very much in its infancy and consequently only a small number of methodological techniques have so far been developed; we can, however, draw on the experiences of those researchers who have worked with other service users who have communication difficulties, such as those with learning difficulties.

COLLECTING THE OPINIONS OF PEOPLE WITH DEMENTIA ON THE SERVICES THAT THEY USE

At least three ways of collecting the opinions of people with dementia directly have so far been described:

- questionnaires and structured interviews
- semi-structured interviews
- focus groups.

Questionnaires/structured interviews

Where the service user with dementia has relatively mild cognitive impairments it may, in some cases, be possible to evaluate services using short questionnaires or structured interviews. Because older people are often unfamiliar with form-filling, many find forms both anxiety-provoking and confusing (Hazell, Driver and Shalan 1996). Consequently, this method is most likely to produce reliable and valid measures of users' views if it is administered personally by the researcher within the service setting being evaluated (Sperlinger and McAuslane 1994). The validity of these forms of evaluation can be enhanced by using clear language, focused questions and visual aids such as photographs.

In their 1994 study Sperlinger and McAuslane found that clients with dementia were rarely interested in commenting on the physical aspects of the service that they received but often focused their comments on its social aspects (for example, other clients and staff). This suggests that the more rigid formats of questionnaires and structured interviews, in which issues for evaluation are set prior to the interview, may not match the concerns of the client group (Murray 1996). It may be that a mixture of either/or, multiple-choice and open-ended questions would enable clients to express not only positive comments but negative feedback as well, as has been the case for people with learning difficulties (Chapman and Oakes 1995). Using these methods enables an evaluation to move from providing a simple measure of satisfaction with the service received to assessing aspects of the service that are failing or that are not currently available but considered desirable by the client.

Semi-structured interviews

As an alternative to the rigid structure of questionnaires it is possible to use a more informal interview procedure in which the interviewer's questions follow a series of general topics, allowing the person with dementia to raise issues not on the original agenda but which may be personally salient for them. Using such semi-structured interviews, Sperlinger and McAuslane (1994) found that all but one of the respondents in their study was able to supply information about themselves and their views of the service. Their experiences led them to suggest interviewing users on more than one occasion and audiotaping the sessions. This allows anxiety which may be present during a first interview to recede and trust between client and researcher to build up. It also enables the researcher to assess whether the clients' views are consistent or changeable.

It is important that the interviews with service users are conducted by a person *not* involved in directly providing the clinical services, as this may well influence the replies (Hazell *et al.* 1996).

The answers of service users, once gathered from the interviews, can then be coded into categories. These categories may arise from the data itself (e.g. through grounded theory – Glaser and Strauss 1967) or may be grouped along pre-existing lines. The content analysis used by Sutton and Fincham

(1994) drew on categories developed for life-planning work with people with learning disabilities.

Jake Smallwood, who worked at the Holyhill Unit in Birmingham, piloted a project which aimed to interview people with dementia about the activities that they participated in and those that they would like to do (Smallwood 1997). In all, he interviewed 11 people from assessment units and a day centre, all of whom had mild to moderate dementia. Each participant was interviewed twice so that it was possible to check whether or not themes and issues from the first interview were repeated. This provided an indication of how reliable the interviews could be considered to be.

Overall, over two-thirds of the issues from the first interview were repeated in the second interview. As there were difficulties with coding some of the material, this figure is probably something of an underestimate, but does indicate that the issues that the dementia sufferers brought up were of lasting significance to them rather than being passing concerns. From this research, Smallwood suggests that working with people in this way raises a number of possibilities for service development, including:

- individualising the services that people receive
- providing them with the opportunity to have some control over the care that they receive
- allowing a quality check
- providing an opportunity for people to express their feelings about the services that they receive
- giving people the chance to express their wishes for the future.

Focus groups

The views of service users can be sought by group discussion (Murray 1996). This enables users to make recommendations to service managers, particularly if given a remit for discussion prior to the meetings. Disadvantages of this method are that it requires a skilled facilitator, and that the views of clients with greater verbal competence are likely to be heard at the expense of others. However, support gained from being with others may enable individuals to express views they would otherwise not verbalise.

EVALUATING SERVICE PROVISION FROM THE PERSPECTIVE OF PEOPLE WITH DEMENTIA

Given the verbal and cognitive deficits of people with dementia, it may sometimes not be possible simply to rely on their memories on issues that concern them. Moreover, patient satisfaction rates are generally very high, regardless of whether or not the patient suffers from a cognitive disability. This is because recipients of services are usually so desperately grateful for whatever service is provided that they feel it would be foolish for them to express their concerns fully – which, in some units, is certainly an accurate perception. Also, they may have little sense of what alternative provision might be possible.

Observation

Observation is a method widely used by researchers working in the area of learning difficulties and is probably the one that has been used most often in dementia care. Observation can be used in a structured way – for example, through Dementia Care Mapping, as we have described above. Alternatively, observation can be used in a more unstructured manner, where the researcher 'shadows' the individual and tries to immerse themselves in the reality of the user's world. A drawback to this method, noted by Barnett (1997), is that there can be a disparity between the 'observed' experience and the way in which dementia sufferers experience the service. An excellent review of observational studies into the quality of care provided for people with dementia living within institutions has been provided by Brooker (1995).

Advocacy

Many service evaluations seek the views of relatives, carers or keyworkers as advocates of service users, even though these figures are not independent sources of service evaluation. Nevertheless, they will often be the people who know the person with dementia best and who are most likely to have an insight into their needs, wishes, likes and dislikes. However, where professional staff are asked to evaluate their own service there is the potential for a conflict of interest. An advocate, by contrast, is someone who either speaks on behalf of a user or facilitates the views of the user themselves. To use advocates effectively in the evaluation of services requires that they be independent of all parties other than the client themselves (Burton 1997).

ETHICAL ISSUES INVOLVED IN HEARING THE VOICE OF DEMENTIA SUFFERERS

There is a range of ethical considerations involved in obtaining the views of people with dementia who use mental health and social services. Included are issues of consent, confidentiality, feedback and meaningful empowerment.

Consent

To ensure that users of services are able to give their consent in a meaningful way, researchers must use every available opportunity to present the rationale for the evaluation. At the same time, it is important to ensure that individuals appreciate that there will be no negative consequences if they chose not to take part or if they chose not to answer all the questions. It is also necessary, at each appointment, to remind participants that they may end an interview at any point.

Confidentiality

The first approach to users of services to gain consent for participation should be through a professional who is already working with the client (Chapman and Oakes 1995). Thereafter, confidentiality must remain the paramount consideration for researchers, with clients' information coded anonymously and information drawn from the evaluation presented in such a manner that individual respondents cannot be recognised.

Feedback

All research involving seeking the views of a given group should entail feedback to that group concerning the findings. While this may seem a difficult task in the field of dementia, logically, feedback should be no more difficult than the data-gathering. After all, the researcher will have had to think how best to gain the information they are interested in from the client. If they can gain information they can surely work out ways of communicating the findings.

Empowerment

Such feedback can aid in empowerment. If we seek to involve dementia sufferers in evaluating the services that they receive through interviews and observation then we have a duty to ensure that this information really makes a difference to the future provision of services. If reliable structures are not in place to ensure that their voice is heard and acted upon, then exercises such as these can be accused of amounting to no more than tokenism.

Changing and improving the service

As the recommendations that are generated by an evaluation will reflect local conditions it is impossible to provide off-the-peg solutions. Instead, we would like to finish this section by outlining a series of questions that can be used when thinking about the sorts of services that you work in.

- *Is your unit maximising the opportunities of its clients to maintain their activities and their networks in the community?* It is all too easy for units to become inward-looking and interested only in what happens *inside* the unit. But the real proof of a unit's quality is how the person interacts outside the unit. Even in residential and nursing homes the importance of going out and maintaining links with the local area cannot be overemphasised. Likewise, relatives need to be made welcome so that their links are maintained; and they need to feel free to take the person out and/or bring friends in. There is rarely, if ever, a good clinical reason why people with dementia should not continue to take part in community activities even after admission to a nursing or residential home.

  All too often, when a person changes from living at home to residential care their attendance at a day centre is stopped. This is done as a cost-saving exercise but justified on the grounds that the residential or nursing home should provide for all aspects of care, occupational included. Even if this were true, which certainly is far from the case, breaking up the person's friendship links with other clients and staff at the day centre is callous and detrimental to their well-being. They have enough to grieve about on losing their independence without having to experience further unnecessary losses.

- *Is your unit providing a secure and trusting structure?* One possible indicator of this is whether patients are able to talk to staff about the experience of being assessed or how they feel about being in the unit or ward, and whether their concerns are taken seriously and acted upon. There should always be a variety of occasions – individual, group, formal and informal – on which concerns can be aired and treated as meaningful and important.

- We believe that *people with mild or moderate dementia can benefit from regular supportive counselling sessions.* Staff should receive training in such skills and each client who *might* benefit should be allocated a weekly time slot. Regardless of whether staff receive counselling training and regardless of the severity of dementia of their clients, staff need training to maximise their understanding of vocal and non-verbal communications from clients and enable them to communicate through those modalities.

- *Is there a clear routine to the day, or is it variable or confusing?* There needs to be a balance between having a clear structure and routine to the day and the sense of there being opportunities for growth and learning. Each day should not be like the last: quite the opposite. Good dementia care should allow people with dementia to take risks and try new tasks – things they are much more likely to do if they feel secure.

- *Can you move the focus of the unit away from the clients' disability – their memory loss – so as to make each day memorable?* In a very nice piece of work, Backman (1992) showed that days on which the clients went on outings were better remembered than ordinary days. In a similar mode, Ikeda *et al.* (1998) (*see also* Williams and Garner 1998), in Japan, have shown that people with dementia remember an earthquake far better than their CAT scan. We realise that it may take a little organisation on your part to achieve either! Nevertheless, this research points to the need to make days distinctive.

- In terms of familiarity, *would the keyworker system and/or small teams who consistently work with an individual be a useful way of working?* If this form of working already exists, do members of teams have the opportunity to go over their work together, to develop care-plans and identify areas of psychological work?

- As a first goal, *can each client participate each week in at least one activity that is particularly relevant to their needs?* And, in a like manner, *can we give each staff member a group or activity which is aimed at helping their development,* so they have one group or activity that they are responsible for?

Turning to the needs of relatives of people who have dementia:

- There will be occasions when, because our primary responsibility is to the client, i.e. the person with dementia, *health and social services and voluntary agencies will need to act as advocates for people with dementia.* This may mean that information is exchanged between client and staff to which relatives have no right of access. An obvious example would be what is talked about in the counselling sessions. We do not think that relatives will have any problem understanding such prioritisation and boundaries if the philosophy of the unit is explained to them at the beginning in a sharing rather than a 'take it or leave it' way.

- At the same time, our commitment to people with dementia means that *services should aim to maintain and support the family systems in which people with dementia live and are cared for.* If our services are to be effective in keeping people with moderate or severe dementia in the community then they must act as a resource for relatives. If we are to do this effectively then it would help to avoid the blanket term 'carer', which has allowed relationships of all shapes and sizes to be squashed into a catch-all. A little reflection helps us to realise that some relatives are soldiering on, others are surviving by keeping a stiff upper lip and buttoning down their emotions, and others are shocked and depressed at what has happened to their loved one. Now if we lump relatives with these varying and various needs into one group and call them 'carers', then we are doing everyone a disservice.

- So, *our services need to develop good lines of communication with the relatives of clients at an individual level* and with relatives' groups such as the ADS, to see how units can be most responsive to them and their needs. We need, therefore, to have a *variety* of ways of helping relatives – individual sessions on request, social support groups, groups for troubled relatives and so on.

To summarise these points, we have stressed often in the last few pages that services for people with dementia should have a primary responsibility and commitment to the sufferers themselves. However, we are fully conscious of the fact that in terms of maintaining systems, *a unit that is being effective in keeping people with moderate or severe dementia in the community must be a resource centre to the relatives and of readily available help to them.*

Concluding this chapter, all these aims – for the person with dementia and for their relatives – should be seen in the wider context of purpose and philosophy. Are we allowing our clients to develop their skills? Are we providing a structure that welcomes risk taking within a stable structure? Are staff pacing their interventions at the right speed to maximise comprehension? *Is this the kind of place I would like a relative of mine to go if they had dementia?*

Summary of main points

- The majority of people with dementia live in the community, either on their own or with relatives. Their standard of living depends to a large extent upon their economic circumstances.
- Although the primary responsibility of services should be to the client – the person with dementia – this orientation need not and should not stop the unit providing individualised support to relatives.

- In order for significant change to be made in the culture of care within an organisation, it is important to try to change the way that the system as a whole operates. It is important to set up systems which have routine evaluation built into them so that areas that need to be improved are identified, appropriate teaching or training can be given and the effects of this training can be monitored.

- Such training may include Dementia Care Mapping and training in counselling, basic listening skills and awareness of the attachment needs of people with dementia.

- Methods of evaluating the impact of care from the perspective of the person with dementia and drawing out the opinions of people with dementia are being developed.

- Solutions must relate to the local situation, although we have also outlined a number of areas of potential development.

- The cycle of change, including careful staff selection, is ongoing. The knowledge and methods are now available to provide high quality care to people with dementia. Not to do so is to make an active decision to be neglectful of them.

PART FOUR

Looking to our Future

CHAPTER 16

Obstacles to Change

Throughout this book we have emphasised that at the heart of dementia care lies the relationship between people with dementia and those who care for them, be they husbands, wives, sons, daughters, nurses, occupational therapists, social workers or psychologists.

There is nothing new in this. What we feel is new is the belief that at their best, these relationships can be and indeed should be therapeutic. Here, we would argue, is the essential difference between the forms of dementia care suggested by the organic model and by the new culture of dementia care. The organic model sees the relationship between a person with dementia and those around him or her as essentially the means to an end – that of helping the person with dementia to attend the local day centre, take their medication or engage in other interactions.

In the person-centred approach described by Tom Kitwood and in the person-focused work that we have outlined here, the process of developing an empathic, supportive relationship is an end in itself. Helping people with dementia to feel secure, to be able to maintain a coherent and positive sense of themselves, to express and understand their emotions – all of this can be seen as being therapeutic, but only if one begins to understand dementia as something more than the loss of brain cells, as something other than simply the degradation of cognitive functioning.

Understanding why the organic model has been so successful

There is a very old 'yokel' joke in which a couple from the city are walking in the countryside and ask a yokel the way to a certain town. He scratches his head and says 'Well if I were you, I wouldn't start from here'. We feel much the same way about dementia care.

This somewhat pessimistic conclusion may seem at odds with the present upbeat state of research. After all, a series of new drugs, 'the cognitive enhancers', are coming on line and there is a huge increase in interest in the social aspects of dementia. New training organisations and university departments have been created to co-ordinate research in this field and new service organisations for people with dementia and their relatives are being set up in many areas.

Yet this success is, paradoxically, part of the problem. Construing dementia as a broad disease category with a number of discrete sub-categories has permitted significant advances in drug design, which seem to have the potential to make a significant impact over the next decade. We have also seen a rapid increase in our knowledge about the genetic and neurological aspects of dementia.

But, as we have argued throughout this book, this can only ever be *part* of the story of dementia. Understanding dementia as an illness in this way does very little to help us to understand how to intervene, how to care for people with dementia or how to talk with them. Indeed, the emphasis on people as dysfunctioning brains has, arguably, contributed significantly to the impoverished care environments that are so often seen around people with dementia.

The drug model, by ascribing primacy to brain conditions is antagonistic to models of *social* change which imply that there is a reality greater than the individual's brain. Moreover, in a culture that is always in a hurry, the much faster relief that drugs offer is of great importance. Medication can offer an apparently quick way to calm people down and lift their mood or to keep a ward seemingly calm and orderly. The fact that many of these drugs have side effects is often played down or ignored. Benzodiazapines, such as Valium and Librium, create a strong dependency if taken for over a period of several months, with patients needing to take ever-increasing and progressively less effective doses. Similarly, anti-psychotic medication can cause organic brain damage if used on a long-term basis, while for older adults there is always an increased risk of side effects. (The reader is referred to Breggin (1993) and Healy (1997) for much more fuller expositions of the damaging effects of psychotrophic drugs.)

If we are to combat the influence of this model, then, we need to understand why it has continued to be so powerful, and why living in the shadow of this model of dementia is so difficult for psychosocial patterns of care. The main reason why we are pessimistic about the possibility of significant, widespread change in dementia care occurring is because the organic model serves many functions for a variety of groups.

The organic model as part of the system of psychiatry

If we look at the history of psychiatry in the 1950s and 1960s, we can see that, broadly speaking, it had two wings – social and organic – that, if not balanced, were at least prepared to acknowledge the other's existence and, albeit grudgingly, give some credence to the alternative point of view. This balance of power changed after the 1970s. As we outlined in chapter 1, the third edition of the *Diagnostic and Statistical Manual* published by the American Psychiatric Association in 1980 represented a concerted push to establish an organic disease model of psychiatry as *the only valid model.*

The advance of organic psychiatry can be seen very clearly in the field of schizophrenia. In the 1960s and 1970s, there were influential theories in the United States – such as Ackerman (1958), Wynne *et al.* (1958) and Bateson *et al.* (1956) – all hypothesising that maladaptive family dynamics had a causal role in an individual developing schizophrenia. In this country, Laing's writings – *The Divided Self* (1959) – especially the later, more popular, ones such as *The Politics of Experience* (1967) were probably the best known expositions of this general perspective.

In the 1980s, more sophisticated medical and biomedical research began, including the use of scans and genetic research. Soon, organic theories of schizophrenia and other psychoses such as manic depression had become dominant within psychiatry. The social context, including the families in which people with schizophrenia live, was seen as important only in determining the chance of relapse into mental illness. Thus, interventions which trained families of a person with schizophrenia to solve their problems together, and which aimed to reduce the amount of stress experienced by the person with schizophrenia, continued to be developed. But despite the apparent effectiveness of these and other psychological and social interventions, the dominant model within which they developed was of drug use and the main focus of research was upon the genetic and neurological mechanisms involved in schizophrenia. (The nature of dementia was seen as so evidently organic that it was not deemed worthy of much discussion.)

These organic explanations have become part of the power and authority of those who have status. To alter the way of thinking about people and their problems, including their mental health problems, is to risk losing this authority. What is true of schizophrenia is doubly true in the field of dementia research.

The organic model and drug companies

Drug companies are very big business. Glaxo-Wellcome, for example, is one of the largest companies in the United Kingdom. Drugs that promise to reduce the symptoms of common conditions, such as arthritis or asthma or alleviate mental illnesses such as schizophrenia or dementia, are all extremely profitable.

As Kirk and Kutchins (1992) show, the relationship between American psychiatry and the drug companies is very close. Research into drug efficacy is undertaken by psychiatrists on behalf of drug companies, while the companies fund research programmes and academic development, travel to conferences and so on. There is a well-established, well-funded network of drug company salespeople all attempting to promote the latest products. The drug companies themselves have a sophisticated strategy of marketing, production and pricing.

Taken overall, if an amount of money equivalent to that spent on medical, genetic and biochemical research was spent on improving living conditions, then this would have a dramatic effect on the frequency of severe mental illness, as many illnesses, including dementia, are related to social class and poorer living conditions (Hollingshead and Redlich 1958; Lindesay et al. 1989). But drug companies, understandably, have no interest in psychosocial research. Their interests lie solely in construing people's problems as illnesses and producing drugs to reduce the effects of these illnesses.

Although, at the time of writing, the first drug licensed for use in the UK to combat the cognitive decline involved in dementia (Aricept) is struggling to be accepted as effective or cost-effective in the NHS (Melzer 1998), it is easy to foresee a time in the not too distant future when similar drugs will be marketed to elderly people who do not have dementia but suffer from what some psychiatrists and others now refer to as 'benign seniscent forgetfulness' (the fall off in memory that can occur in old age) and even to school and university students who need help with their exams.

The organic model as a means of coping

The power of the organic model does not just stem from psychiatry and the drug companies. It serves an important function for both people with demen- tia and their relatives. As we have argued throughout this book, people with dementia and their relatives need to know what is happening without this knowledge being so overwhelming that they feel submerged and lost. Explanations which focus on an illness can allow them to manage the knowledge that something is wrong without feeling either personally responsible or completely lost. After all, most people have much experience of being 'ill' and of doctors and nurses curing and caring for us.

Holding on to the idea of oneself and one's relatives as being ill, then, is part of the coping strategy that some people with dementia use and which we outlined in Part Two of this book. Their relatives, too, will often be comforted by such an explanation. In many ways, it is easier to see the illness as solely a neurological problem than to think of the person with dementia as still existing as a mental and social being with awareness and insight, in an interpersonal network.

In the context of huge and varied drug use, the use of a drug to achieve a given state – be it recovering from the loss of a partner, getting back to work when you have flu or getting your memory back – seems a perfectly reasonable thing to do. There is a widespread social expectation that if there is a problem a drug can cure it. For many people with dementia and their relatives, the understandable expectation is that there will soon be a cure for dementia, even though the best that can so far be offered is a temporary delay in the rate at which symptoms progress. The organic model holds out hope for people – the hope that soon all of the agony and despair will be reduced, that a magic pill will arrive.

An additional function of the organic model for relatives is that it helps to assuage *carer guilt*. Whenever we or a person we care for become ill or disabled, we seek an explanation. One type of explanation that many people arrive at is that their own behaviour caused the condition (e.g. 'If I hadn't worked so hard, I wouldn't have had the heart attack'; 'If I had been there, she wouldn't have fallen over and broken her hip'). Explanations based on the organic model help to transform personal relationships and their breakdown into a breakdown in the patient's neurological functioning. What *should* happen (but rarely does) is that good counselling be made available to help relatives to work through their fears and irrational self-blame.

Finally, the over-pathologising of a condition such as learning disability, schizophrenia or dementia serves another function. Imagine trying to run a fund-raising campaign on the platform: 'Dementia is an uncommon illness. Some people with dementia will become aggressive, but most won't, and many will die before their condition becomes very severe – so please give generously'. Instead the message is much more likely to be along the lines of 'all people with dementia will inevitably deteriorate, and that includes you if you're unfortunate enough to get it, which is a distinct likelihood. So please give generously'. As we described in Chapter 1, the re-creation of Alzheimer's disease as the main form of dementia rather than as an obscure form of pre-senile dementia, as it had previously been taken to be, was driven in part by a concern to facilitate raising funds for research.

Of course, this kind of campaigning has a horrible drawback. If dementia inevitably leads to terminal decline then interventions (and certainly psychosocial intervention) are not useful. Thus, staff training is necessary, but only to meet the physical needs of patients, and the number of staff can be kept to a minimum. When, on some occasions, we are called into units with little interest in social care to advise on a client's aggressive behaviour, we cannot help wondering if the pawn in this game is expressing their anger at one too many insult or one too many occasion of neglect.

The social functions of the organic model

The organic model also serves a series of functions for society at large. Gubrium (1986), for instance, has suggested that underlying the familiar differentiation of an 'abnormal' old age (dementia) from a 'normal' old age is a wish to see certain of the symptoms of ageing as symptoms of a disease, and hence as being potentially curable. The process whereby images of decay have been transformed into images of disease represents part of the symbolic change that we, as a society, have made to remove ageing from the realm of nature and place it within the realm of science. Through this transformation, we can hope for a cure and hence the prevention of our own decay.

The severe devaluation of people with dementia can also be seen as separating the untouchables from the rest of society. The key denial in dementia is therefore that of society. The construction of dementia as a discrete process, as something that happens to some people but not to others, serves to distance all of us from the human tragedy involved in 'losing one's mind' (Sutton 1994). Construing dementia simply in terms of a disease of the brain means that personal challenges can be more easily avoided.

The organic model and private nursing and residential homes

There is another major group among whom the organic model has become established – private nursing and residential homes. A major feature of care for older people over the last 20 years has been the transference of responsibility for long-term care from the NHS to the private sector. Partly in response to the financial need to reduce bed numbers and increase bed turnover, and partly because of the emphasis on the policy of community care, much of the NHS has moved from providing long-term or continuing care for people with dementia to providing beds only for assessment and respite care.

If the philosophy of the new culture of dementia care is to become part of the culture of these private nursing homes then a range of issues must be addressed. These include the low numbers of staff, especially trained staff, their poor pay and prospects, the dearth of structured activity for residents and the often low standard of psychological care. The only organisation with sufficient political clout to insist on the necessary changes is central government, through the current system of registration and the regular inspection of homes by registration officers. At present, registration is almost completely confined to relatively easily measured aspects of the physical care environment; the social quality of care is simply not addressed.

Clearly, a major factor acting against central government insisting on a higher quality of psychosocial care are the cost implications of such a move, since it would involve the need for more and better qualified staff. But one source might be the NHS. With dementia we have the odd situation that the NHS has relatively few beds but most of the trained nurses, psychologists and physiotherapists etc., while the residential and nursing homes have most of the beds but few of the trained staff.

Clearly, the situation is unbalanced. However, it can only become balanced by government action which values people with dementia enough to increase funding to the Social Service departments which finance many of these beds. Otherwise, the pitiful neglect of people with dementia will continue indefinitely.

The organic model and purchasers of services

Above all else, if the new culture is to have a significant impact, then there needs to be significantly more investment in the people who will make it work. Work with people with dementia can be 1:3 in the early stages. After that, it has to be much more intensive, with staffing ratios of 1:2 or 1:1½ if effective relationships are to be possible. Few staffing levels in day hospitals, nursing homes or elsewhere approach anything like this level. Moreover, work with people with dementia requires *more* skill, not less, than work with people who do not have cognitive loss. We need staff with good individual counselling and groupwork skills who receive regular supervision.

Dementia care will *not* improve until we have enough competent staff, and this requires a level of commitment from managers and purchasers that has so far been lacking. Talk to any social worker working with the elderly and they will tell you how their assessment of needs must be 'realistic', i.e. within financial constraints. Each year, these financial constraints seem to become fiercer and so the services that can be offered become fewer and for shorter periods. Above all else, this lack of managerial and financial clout is perhaps the main reason to fear that the new culture of dementia care will fail to make the impact that is so widely hoped for.

Summary of main points

- The organic model has produced much of great importance, including drugs that can enhance the cognitive functioning of dementia sufferers. However, understanding people with dementia simply as dysfunctional brains is of limited use for day-to-day dementia care.

- The organic model exists because it serves many functions for a variety of social groupings, from people with dementia themselves to international drug company conglomerates, and, in a wider setting, society itself.

- If we are really going to try to introduce a new culture of dementia care we need a high staff ratio and, in particular, a good number of trained staff who have individual and groupwork skills. Because of the nature of these functions and the financial commitment that it would take to implement the forms of change that we believe are necessary, we are pessimistic about the possibility of widespread and significant change occurring in dementia care practices.

CHAPTER 17

Producing Change
A Restless Farewell

We realise that the last chapter makes somewhat depressing reading, but feel that it is important that the reader has the information they need to make sense of the larger picture.

As we set out in the last chapter, we do see major difficulties in achieving individualised quality care for people with dementia. We are worried about whether there is sufficient political and professional interest to support such a goal. At present there seems to be little prospect of people with dementia moving high enough up the professional and political agendas to make this possible.

How, then, can individual mental health workers try to achieve change within their own services? We will end this book with a few suggestions.

Trying to achieve change

The first step in trying to achieve change is to be realistic and tell it how it is. In some ways this could be thought to be an exciting time in dementia research. After all, new ideas have been discussed and many people working in the field have high ideals. Certainly, there are plenty of quotations that we can use to show how many distinguished authors have represented this as an exciting time. For instance:

> The new culture of dementia care is a very exciting one.
> (Marshall 1996, p.2)

> Working with people with dementia and their carers must be the most exciting field of social work to be in at the moment ... Why is it all so new and exciting? (Chapman and Marshall 1993, pp.1–3)

The old culture is one of domination, technique, evasion and buck-passing. To enter the new culture is like coming home. We can now draw close to other human beings, accepting all we genuinely share. (Kitwood and Benson 1995, p.11)

There is, however, an important respect in which thinking of this as an excit-ing time is misleading and, indeed, even counterproductive. Trying to achieve change involves playing the long game, as change of the magnitude that is required cannot be achieved in the short term. Senior managers pin mission statements on the wall, but it is on the floor of the units that the many small decisions that improve dementia care are made by the staff. The day-to-day experience of people working in dementia care is rarely, if ever, exciting – far more often it is one of frustration, boredom and exasperation. When you are trying to achieve change it is all too easy to shut off when faced with such huge difficulties, to close down and acquiesce with the levels of current provision and be left feeling guilty at one's inability to achieve change.

So, how can we make things better, giving ourselves a chance to succeed, without burning ourselves out in the process?

To borrow a phrase from ecologists: 'think global, act local'

We need to hang on to the big picture – the need to change services as a whole – while realising that the only way to do this is to make small changes to our local services. We need to be realistic about the amount of change that can occur and the speed at which we can produce it.

By networking, so that you are working with/sharing ideas with/gaining support from like-minded others

Trying to achieve change on one's own is very lonely. Not only is it difficult to maintain your integrity but, as a lone voice, you can be very vulnerable to marginalisation, if not dismissal. Identifying potential allies is vital – know-ing others value your ideas becomes very important to the maintenance of your beliefs and sanity (Georgiades and Phillimore 1975). Obviously, face-to-face contacts and meetings will help most and be most fruitful, but other forms of communication such as e-mail may augment the process.

By experimenting with ideas and methods without worrying about only using ideas which have been proven through research. We need to experiment wisely but experiment all the same

In the last few years there has been increasing pressure for all activities in which health and welfare professionals engage to be for specific purposes. So, for instance, one of the authors has to record what they are doing every 15 minutes of their working day, and that activity must be within a range of agreed activities and purchased through a specific contract. This might seem an eminently rational way of monitoring an expensive and fairly scarce resource (clinical psychology time) until you realise that it severely limits the clinician's capacity to play with ideas, to be curious and to experiment – that is to say, to be creative.

Working in a loose grouping of people looking at ways of developing ideas and methods is a much freer way of being and thinking than depending on established research methodologies. We need to emphasise the importance of unstructured time spent sharing ideas as part of maintaining professional health.

By pooling research ideas and methods

In order to achieve change it is often necessary to substantiate claims made for the impact of any new service developed. These changes can be bolstered by hard evidence, making it harder for changes to be reversed. This means that we need to engage in evaluation and in research. However, research requirements are necessarily high and stringent. Because of the focus on service delivery and speed of delivery, the mental health practitioner is using existing knowledge and is not necessarily in a good position to develop or to evaluate new methods. (Contrast this situation with the millions of pounds available to develop new drugs and to do the background research to develop new understandings of how the body and brain works in order to facilitate the development of drugs.)

Given, then, the very limited time and opportunity to undertake research, it is very difficult for an individual practitioner to undertake it on their own. However, by pooling research ideas and methods, a sufficient sample size can be achieved across, say, four or six sites. Research into psychotherapy with people with dementia, for instance, may need to occur within looser configurations and with greater co-operation with colleagues in other areas and fields than is often the case. It may also need to proceed without significant research funding, as this tends to be available only to traditional forms of work and traditional research methodologies.

What we are hoping could be achieved by the above suggestions is that:

1. a larger number of practitioners undertake individual and group therapy with people who have dementia

2. this effort will not be just with people in the 'early stages' of dementia but with people with dementia of all levels of severity, which means that

3. the exact methods used in therapy will vary greatly from traditional verbal therapy to methods using other modalities such as touch, smell, music and so on

4. this larger number of practitioners will gather such evidence as they can about how and when a given approach is useful, without trying to force it into a strict research methodology.

By focusing on the person with dementia living in the community

Elsewhere in this book we have commented on how much of the clinical research with people with dementia, for instance Reality Orientation, Reminiscence and Validation/Resolution Therapy, has focused on older people living with dementia in institutions. This focus is inevitably unbalanced, ignoring those people with dementia living in their own homes. This latter group of people with dementia tend to be more able, younger and, importantly, less likely to be undergoing the sorts of crisis often found among an institutionalised population.

Focusing instead on people with dementia living in the community would:

- look at where the majority of people with dementia live – their environments and ecologies, both physical and personal
- bring the professional into contact with people who have shorter histories of dementia, whose concern and needs are often substantially different from other people with dementia.

While it would be unrealistic – if not completely misleading – to think in terms of a 'cure' for dementia, what it may be possible to do, by intervening at this early stage, is give the person with dementia a wider and more effective range of skills with which to cope with the difficulties that lie ahead. Generally, such a focus on people with dementia living in the community rather than in institutions must inevitably be more optimistic. This optimism could be transferred into more ambitious therapeutic programmes aimed at primary rather than secondary or tertiary care.

To help the 'young-old' stop denying their ageing and see their community of purpose with the 'old-old'

Finally, if we are going to achieve meaningful change, then we need to alter the political homeostasis that keeps people with dementia at the bottom of the list of priorities. The most effective way to do this would be to engage the 'young-old' in political activity. By 'young-old' we are roughly talking about people between 60 and 75, but, more specifically, we are concerned with people of reasonable physical health and mobility. These people are often very active in community and political organisations – they are people of energy with a spending power to match.

In many ways, the major obstacles to engaging this population are psychological. At four in the morning, they turn over in bed and know that their spouse and friends will probably die in the next few years, that they will be increasingly alone, and their own health and mobility will decrease, as will their spending power. Such frightening thoughts are best put away in the morning light. This is political suicide, because it means that the one (potential) power group that could change the political balance and get a better deal for the frail elderly – themselves in a few years' time – deliberately turns away from that task.

One of us recently heard two mental health professionals talking at a conference the other day. 'Of course', one said, 'our generation will never put up with conditions in nursing homes, as they now are, when our turn comes – so there are bound to be changes'. The other nodded in agreement.

These thoughts are such pleasant, protective delusions! When they, and we, are 75, there is unlikely to be any more choice about nursing homes than there is now. Like a 75-year-old today, some major aspect of their and our skills and physical well-being will have gone. So, unless they and we have engaged in some political activity long before that time comes, the nursing home they and we go to will be much like the ones that they and we visit professionally today.

Keeping people in the community does not need therapists and it does not need magic. It needs money and resources, so that people are able to move around and keep up their activities and friendships. It also needs resources such as home care, meals-on-wheels etc. to support and do the things that people with dementia cannot do. We require the resources to help caring relatives from becoming overstretched and exhausted. What is needed for people with dementia is what is needed for people with any type of disability. Indeed, it is what all older people who have limited resources need. So, there is no great mystery – just a political reluctance to give older people in general, and people with dementia in particular, the priority that they need and deserve.

One of the most effective ways to move dementia up the funding ladder would be for the young-old to begin to ask searching questions about the quality of care available to people with dementia at both national and local levels. Single-illness organisations are not in the best position to do so, as their constituents are by definition already disabled. For instance, people joining the Alzheimer's Disease Society already have a relative with dementia. A goodly proportion will probably be old-old themselves (i.e. 75+) and not in the best of health, and so are unlikely to have the time and energy to pursue a political agenda. It requires larger organisations with a broader interest in the needs of all older people – Age Concern, for instance – to take a lead. Perhaps even such organisations are seen as too stigmatising by the young-old. Perhaps a new, more politically- rather than welfare-focused organisation or grouping will also be needed.

We know that political priorities – and the access to resources that goes with them – can change. Perhaps the most successful refusal to accept second rate services was achieved by people who were HIV+ or had AIDS. They achieved the ring-fencing of resources for those conditions and almost no discussion about the cost of treatment. Other pressure groups have also had their successes: MIND has fought to protect and maintain the legal rights of people with severe mental illnesses; people with learning difficulties and their advocates have successfully fought for small units in the community to replace the large mental handicap hospitals; and people with physical disabilities have fought for access to public buildings and equal opportunities.

So positive change and improvements in standards for disabled groups is both possible and achievable. But, in contrast, older people with dementia are on low pensions and if they cannot stay in the community then they must go into large nursing homes. As professionals, we therefore need to improve our political performance – and our natural allies in seeking to improve the conditions of people with dementia are the young-old.

The young-old, with their post-retirement health, energy and income, have the numbers and the potential clout to improve conditions for the old-old, including those with dementia. Acting now would improve conditions for themselves in the years to come. It would also improve conditions for us and for you, the reader, a little further down the line.

The psychologist liked to follow up people he had assessed in order to see the longitudinal patterns.

The man who gave this book its title died about four years after the assessment at the age of 72 years. His widow, and one of his daughters who was present, told of how, in his last months, his balance had been severely affected and his speech reduced to the occasional 'Yes' and, less frequently, 'No'. Because of his difficulties with balance, his wife was unable to cope and he spent his last few months in a nursing home, being visited daily by his family.

Death and the passage of time had allowed a return to an understanding of his whole life and his considerable achievement across its span.

At the end of the interview, as the psychologist rose to leave, the daughter said sadly 'Because he spoke so little in the last few months, I can't remember the sound of Dad's voice.'

Further Reading

The following books might be of help to you in understanding psychosocial ideas applied to the field of dementia:

Nancy Harding and Colin Palfrey (1997) *The Social Construction of Dementia: Confused Professionals?* London: Jessica Kingsley Publishers.
A difficult read but a well-argued account of how 'dementia' has been socially constructed as a disease.

Tom Kitwood and Sue Benson (eds) (1995) *The New Culture of Dementia Care.* London: Hawker Publications.
The book – a collection of papers – that announced the arrival of 'the new culture of dementia care' based on the work of Kitwood's unit at Bradford University.

Tom Kitwood (1997) *Dementia Reconsidered: The Person Comes First.* Buckingham: Open University Press.
A bringing together and updating of Kitwood's pioneering papers of the late 1980s and early 1990s on the need to apply a psychological perspective to dementia. This book won the 1998 Age Concern Book of the Year prize.

Accounts of the personal experience of dementia:

Louis Blank (1995) *Alzheimer's Challenged and Conquered?* London: Foulsham.
Some critics have doubted that this highly intelligent man, living in his council flat in Rochdale, ever had Alzheimer's, but his psychiatrist so diagnosed him and Blank describes how he found his way out.

Robert Davis (1989) *My Journey into Alzheimer's Disease.* Buckingham: Scriptured Press.
There was no way out for this highly successful priest. His fight against his feelings of betrayal by God and his account (helped by his wife) of the loss of his skills is absolutely harrowing.

Diana McGowin (1993) *Living in the Labyrinth*. Cambridge: Mainsail Press.
This lady is feisty. Although quite damaged by the end of her account, she makes it clear that she'll go down fighting.

Carer accounts:

Lore K. Wright (1993) *Alzheimer's Disease and Marriage*. Newsbury Park: Sage.
A straight research study of 30 couples, one of whom had Alzheimer's. What makes it relevant is the author's determined attempt to get the views of both members of the marriage.

Margaret Forster (1989) *Have the Men had Enough?* London: Penguin.
The mother starts to dement. The daughters start to quarrel over how she should be cared for. Her end in a home is mind-shrivellingly painful.

Michael Ignatieff (1993) *Scar Tissue*. London: Chatto and Windus.
A fictional account of his mother's change from skilled painter to person with severe dementia. The first part, in which he describes this change and his reactions, is painfully recalled.

Bernard Heywood (1994) *Caring for Maria*. Dorset: Element.
Unlike Forster's fictional account of the effects on the relative of caring over a long period, this is a factual account of how the author becomes involved in caring over many months for his neighbour. The drudgery, exhaustion and loss are all too evident.

References

Ackerman, N.W. (1958) *The Psychodynamics of Family Life*. New York: Basic Books.

Adelman, R.C. (1995) 'The Alzheimerization of aging.' *Gerontologist, 35*, 526–532.

Adshead, F., Cody, D.D. and Pitt, B. (1992) 'BASDEC: A novel screening instrument for depression in elderly medical inpatients.' *British Journal of Psychiatry, 305*, 397.

Agbayewa, M.O. (1986) 'Earlier psychiatric morbidity in patients with Alzheimer's disease.' *Journal of American Geriatric Society, 34*, 8, 561–564.

Ainsworth, M. *et al.* (1978) *Patterns of Attachment: A Psychobiological Study of the Strange Situation*. Hillsdale, NJ: Erlbaum.

Allen, N.H.P. and Burns, A. (1995) 'The non-cognitive features of dementia.' *Reviews in Clinical Gerontology, 5*, 57–75.

Alzheimer, A. (1907) 'über eine eigenartige Erkrankung der Hirnrinde.' *Allgemeine Zeitschrift für Psychiatrie und Psychisch-Gerichtliche Medizin, 64*, 146–148. In English: Alzheimer, A. (1977) 'A unique illness involving the cerebral cortex.' In D.A. Rottenberg and F.H. Hochberg (eds) *Neurological Classics in Modern Translation*. New York: Hafner Press.

Alzheimer, A. (1911) 'Uber eine eigenartige krankheitsfälle des späteren Alters.' *Zeit. gesamte. Neurol. Psychiat., 4*, 356–385.

Alzheimer, A. (1977) 'A unique illness involving the cerebral cortex.' In D.A. Rottenberg and F.H. Hochberg (eds) *Neurological Classics in Modern Translation*. New York: Hafner Press.

Alzheimer's Disease Society (1995) *Right From the Start: Primary Health Care and Dementia*. Report by the Alzheimer's Disease Society, London.

Amaducci, L.A., Rocca, W.A. and Schoenberg, B.S. (1986) 'Original of the distinction between Alzheimer's disease and senile dementia: How history can clarify nosology.' *Neurology, 36*, 1497–1499.

American Psychiatric Association (1980) *Diagnostic and Statistical Manual of Mental Disorders* (3rd ed). Washington DC: American Psychiatric Association.

American Psychiatric Association (1994) *Diagnostic and Statistical Manual of Mental Disorders* (4th edn). Washington DC: American Psychiatric Association.

Ames, D., Ashby, D., Mann, A.H. and Graham, N. (1988) 'Psychiatric illness in elderly residents of Part III homes in one London borough: Prognosis and review.' *Age and Ageing, 17*, 249–256.

Amster, L.B. and Krauss, T. (1974) 'The relationships between life crises and mental deterioration in old age.' *International Journal of Ageing and Human Development, 5*, 51–55.

Annerstedt, L. (1994) 'An attempt to determine the impact of group living care in comparison to traditional long-term care on demented elderly patients.' *Aging Clinical Exp. Res. 6*, 5, 372–380.

Anthony, J.C., Leresche, L., Niaz, U., Von Korff, M.R. and Folstein, M.F. (1982) 'Limits of the "Mini-Mental State" as a screening test for dementia and delirium among hospital patients.' *Psychological Medicine, 12,* 397–408.

Aschaffenburg (1911) *Handbuch der Psychiatrie.* 12 volumes. Leipzig: Deuticke.

Backman, L. (1992) 'Memory training and memory improvement in Alzheimer's disease: Rules and exceptions.' *Acta Neurologica Scandinavica, Supplement, 139,* 84–89.

Baddeley, A. (1986) *Working Memory.* Oxford: Oxford University Press.

Badger, F., Cameron, E. and Evers, H. (1990) 'Waiting to be served/slipping through the net.' *Health Service Journal,* 11 Jan/18 Jan 54–55, 86–87.

Bahro, M., Silber, E., Box, P. and Sunderland, T. (1995) 'Giving up driving in Alzheimer's disease: An integrative therapeutic approach.' *International Journal of Geriatric Psychiatry, 10,* 871–874.

Balfour, A. (1995) 'Account of a study aiming to explore the experience of dementia.' *PSIGE Newsletter,* No. 53, July, 15–19.

Barnett, E. (1997) 'Listening to people with dementia and their carers.' In M. Marshall (1997) (ed) *State of the Art in Dementia Care.* London: Centre for Policy on Ageing.

Barrowclough, C. and Tarrier, N. (1997) *Families of Schizophrenic Patients.* Cheltenham: Thornes.

Bartolome, M. and Fernandez, V. (1995) 'Neuropsychological performance – age, education and sex.' *Psicothema, 7,* 1, 105–112.

Barton, R. (1959) *Institutional Neurosis.* Bristol: Wright (3rd edition 1976).

Bateson, G., Jackson, D.D., Haley, J. and Weakland, J. (1956) 'Toward a theory of schizophrenia.' *Behavioural Science, 1,* 251–264.

Bayer, R. (1981) *Homosexuality and American Psychiatry: The Politics of Diagnosis.* New York: Basic.

Bayles, K.A., Tomoeda, C.K. and Trosset, M.W. (1993) 'Alzheimer's disease: Effects on language.' *Developmental Neuropsychology, 9,* 2, 131–160.

Beach, T.G. (1987) 'The history of Alzheimer's disease: Three debates.' *Journal of the History of Medicine and Allied Sciences, 42,* 327–349.

Beard, C., Kokmen, E., Offord, K. and Kurland, L. (1992) 'Lack of association between Alzheimer's disease and education, occupation, marital status or living arrangement.' *Neurology, 42,* 11, 2063–2068.

Beck, A.T. (1976) *Cognitive Therapy and the Emotional Disorders.* Harmondsworth, Middlesex: Penguin.

Benbow, S.M., Marriott, A., Morley, M. and Walsh, S. (1993) 'Family therapy and dementia: Review and clinical experience.' *International Journal of Geriatric Psychiatry, 8,* 717–725.

Bender, M.P. (1993) 'The unoffered chair: The history of therapeutic disdain toward people with learning difficulty.' *Clinical Psychology Forum,* April, 54, 7–12.

Bender, M.P. (1995) 'Orientation by season.' *Nursing Times,* May 2, 64–65.

Bender, M.P. (1996a) *The Man with the Worried Eyes: Researching the Experience of Dementia.* Paper given at a conference of the National Graduate Psychologists' Group, June 22, Manchester Metropolitan University.

Bender, M.P. (1996b) *Listen to the Soft Music of the Triangles.* President's address to the Plymouth Branch of the Alzheimer's Disease Society, 25th July.

Bender, M.P. (1996c) 'Memory clinics: Locked doors on the gravy train?' *PSIGE Newsletter*, October, 58, 30–33.

Bender, M.P. (1997a) *40 Miles of bad road: An account of the strange but true history of the condition or conditions named after Dr Alois Alzheimer.* Paper given to the British Gerontological Society, Plymouth, 13th March.

Bender, M.P. (1997b) 'Bitter harvest: The implications of war-related stress on reminiscence theory and practice.' *Ageing and Society, 17,* 337–348.

Bender, M.P. (1998a) 'Shifting our focus from brain to mind.' *Journal of Dementia Care,* January/February, 6, 1, 20–22.

Bender, M.P. (1998b) *What Happens When You Stop Using the Concept of 'Dementia'? A Post-disease Approach.* Paper given to the Gerontological Research Network Seminar, Southampton University, 12th November.

Bender, M.P. and Bauckham, P. (1998) 'Adapting Reminiscence for the very seriously disoriented.' In Pam Schweitzer (ed) *Reminiscence in Dementia Care.* Blackheath, London: Age Exchange.

Bender, M.P., Bauckham, P. and Norris, A. (1999) *The Therapeutic Uses of Reminiscence.* London: Sage.

Bender, M.P. and Cheston, R. (1997) 'Inhabitants of a lost kingdom: A model of the subjective experiences of dementia.' *Ageing and Society, 17,* 513–532.

Bender, M.P. and Corry, H. (1995) 'Would listening to people with ?dementia be useful?' *PSIGE Newsletter,* 54, October, 25–32.

Bender, M.P., Horrocks, J. and Bullock, T. (1997) *Searching the subjective world of people with dementia.* Paper presented at the UK Dementia Research Group Meeting, Bristol, 27th February.

Bender, M. and Horton, V. (1999) *Where Women Meet: The Exploration of Lives to Increase Understanding of Self, Gender and Disability, Especially Dementia.* To be published.

Bender, M.P., Landers, G., Horrocks, J. and Jones, M. (1999) The Companions Club. *Journal of Dementia Care,* January/February, 28–30.

Bender, M.P., Landers, G., Jones, M. and Kennedy, L. (1999) 'The Companions' Club.' *Journal of Dementia Care,* March/April, 24–25.

Bender, M.P., Levens, V. and Goodson, C. (1995) *Welcoming Your Clients.* Bicester: Winslow.

Bender, M.P. and Wainwright, A. (1998a) *A Model of the Mind in Dementia.* Paper given at the Annual Conference of the Psychologists' Special Interest Group in the Elderly, Napier University, Edinburgh, 2 July.

Bender, M.P. and Wainwright, A. (1998b) 'Dementia: Reversing out of the dead end.' *PSIGE Newsletter 66,* October, 22–25.

Bentall, R. (1990) *Reconstructing Schizophrenia.* Routledge: London.

Bentall, R., Higson, P. and Lowe, C. (1987) 'Teaching self-instruction to schizophrenic patients: Efficacy and generalisation.' *Behavioural Psychotherapy, 15,* 58–76.

Bentall, R., Jackson, H. and Pilgrim, D. (1988) 'Abandoning the concept of "schizophrenia": Some implications of validity arguments for psychological research into psychotic phenomena.' *The British Journal of Clinical Psychology, 27,* 303–324.

Berrios, G.E. (1990) 'Alzheimer's disease: A conceptual history.' *International Journal of Geriatric Psychiatry, 5*, 355–365.

Berrios, G.E. and Brook, P. (1985) 'Delusions and the psychopathology of the elderly with dementia.' *Acta Psychiatrica Scandinavica, 72*, 296–307.

Berrios, G.E. and Freeman, H.L. (eds) (1991) *Alzheimer and the Dementias.* London: Royal Society of Medicine Services.

Berzonsky, M.D. (1990) 'Self-construction over the life span: A process perspective on identity formation.' In G.J. Neimeyer and R.A. Neimeyer (eds) *Advances in Personal Construct Psychology*, Volume 1. Greenwich, Connecticut: Jai Press.

Blank, L. (1995) *Alzheimer's Challenged and Conquered?* London: Foulsham.

Bleathman, C. and Morton, I. (1992) 'Validation therapy: Extracts from 20 groups with dementia sufferers.' *Journal of Advanced Nursing, 17*, 658–666.

Blessed, G., Tomlinson, B.E. and Roth, M. (1968) 'The association between quantative measures of dementia and of senile changes in the cerebral grey matter of elderly subjects.' *British Journal of Psychiatry, 114*, 797–811.

Bleuler, E. (1950) *Dementia Praecox or the Group of Schizophrenias.* New York: International Universities Press. First published 1911.

Bonaiuto, S., Rocca, W., Lippi, A., Giannandrea, E., Mele, M., Cavarzeran, F. and Amaducci, L. (1995) 'Education and occupation as risk factors for dementia – a population based case-control study.' *Neurology, 14*, 3, 101–109.

Bonder, B. (1994) 'Psychotherapy for individuals with Alzheimer's disease.' *Alzheimer's Disease and Associated Disorders, 8*, 3, 75–81.

Bonfiglio, F. (1908) 'Di speciali reperti in un caso di probabile sifilide cerebrale.' *Riv. Sper. Freniatria, 34*, 196–206.

Borch-Jacobsen, M. (1996) *Remembering Anna O.: A Century of Mystification.* New York: Routledge.

Bowlby, J. (1972) *Attachment and Loss: Volume 1: Attachment* (2nd edition). Harmondsworth, Middlesex: Penguin. First published 1969.

Bowlby, J. (1975) *Attachment and Loss, Volume 2: Separation, Anxiety and Anger.* Harmondworth, Middlesex: Penguin.

Bowlby, J. (1981) *Attachment and Loss, Volume 3: Loss: Sadness and Depression.* Harmondworth, Middlesex: Penguin.

Boyle, M. (1990) *Schizophrenia: A Scientific Delusion.* London: Routledge.

Bradford Dementia Group (1997a) *Dementia Care Mapping Manual – 7th edition.* Bradford Dementia Group, University of Bradford.

Bradford Dementia Group (1997b) *Profiling Well-being and Ill-being.* Bradford Dementia Group, University of Bradford.

Bradford Dementia Group (1998) *Dementia Care Mapping: 8th edition.* Bradford University: Bradford Dementia Group.

Breggin, P. (1993) *Toxic Psychiatry.* London: Harper Collins.

Breuer, J. and Freud, S. (1955) 'Studies on hysteria.' In J. Strachey (ed) *Studies in Hysteria. The standard edition of the Complete Psychological Works of Sigmund Freud.* Volume 2. London: Hogarth. First published 1895.

Brody, E.M., Kleban, M.H., Lawton, M.P. and Silverman, H.A. (1971) 'Excess disabilities of mentally impaired aged: Impact of individualised treatment.' *The Gerontologist, 11*, Part 1, 124–133.

Bromley, D.B. (1990) *Behavioural Gerontology: Central Issues in the Psychiatry of Ageing.* Chichester: Wiley.

Brooker, D. (1995) 'Looking at them, looking at me. A review of observational studies into the quality of institutional care for elderly people with dementia.' *Journal of Mental Health, 4,* 145–156.

Brotchie, J., Brennan, J. and Wyke, M.A. (1985) 'Temporal orientation in the pre-senium and old age.' *British Journal of Psychiatry, 147,* 692–695.

Brown, G.W. (1985) 'The discovery of expressed emotion: Induction or deduction.' In J. Leff and C. Vaughn (eds) *Expressed Emotion in Families.* New York: Guildford.

Brown, G.W. and Harris, T. (1978) *Social Origins of Depression.* London: Tavistock.

Brown, H. and Smith, H. (eds) (1992) *Normalisation – A Reader for the Nineties.* London: Tavistock/Routledge.

Buber, M. (1958) *I and Thou* (2nd revised edition). Edinburgh: T. & T. Clark.

Buchanan, K. and Middleton, D. (1993) 'Discursively formulating the significance of reminiscence in later life.' In N. Coupland and J.F. Nussbaum (eds) *Discourse and Lifespan Development.* London: Sage.

Buchanan, K. and Middleton, D. (1994) 'Reminiscence reviewed: A discourse analytic perspective.' In J. Bornat (ed) *Reminiscence Reviewed: Perspectives, Evaluations, Achievements.* Buckingham: Open University.

Buchanan, K. and Middleton, D. (1995) 'Voices of experience: Talk, identity and membership in reminiscence groups.' *Ageing and Society, 15,* 457–491.

Burningham, S. (1992) 'Good practice: Specialist support groups – USA.' *Alzheimer's Disease Society Newsletter.* February.

Burns, A., Howard, R. and Petit, W.C. (1995) *Alzheimer's Disease: A Medical Companion.* Oxford: Blackwell.

Burns, A., Jacoby, R. and Levy, R. (1990a) 'Psychiatric phenomena in Alzheimer's disease I: Disorders of thought content.' *British Journal of Psychiatry, 157,* 72–76.

Burns, A., Jacoby, R. and Levy, R. (1990b) 'Psychiatric phenomena in Alzheimer's Disease II: Disorders of Perception.' *British Journal of Psychiatry, 157,* 76–81.

Burns, A., Jacoby, R. and Levy, R. (1990c) 'Psychiatric phenomena in Alzheimer's Disease III: Disorders of Mood.' *British Journal of Psychiatry, 157,* 81–86.

Burns, A., Jacoby, R. and Levy, R. (1990d) 'Psychiatric phenomena in Alzheimer's Disease IV: Disorders of Behaviour.' *British Journal of Psychiatry, 157,* 86–94.

Burton, A. (1997) 'Dementia: A case for advocacy?' In S. Hunter (ed) *Dementia: Challenges and New Directions.* London: Jessica Kingsley Publishers.

Bury, M. and Holme, A. (1991) *Life After Ninety.* London: Routledge.

Butler, R. (1963) 'The life review: An interpretation of reminiscence in the aged.' *Psychiatry, 26,* 65–76.

Byatt, S. and Cheston, R. (1999) 'Simulated Presence Therapy: A case study.' *Journal of Dementia Care* (to be published).

Bytheway, W. (1995) *Ageism.* Buckingham: Open University.

Canstatt, C.F. (1839) *Der Krankheilen des höheren Alters und ihre Heiling.* Two volumes. Erlangen: Ferninand Enke.

Challis, D., Von Abendorff, R., Brown, P. and Chesterman, J. (1997) 'Care management and dementia: An evaluation of the Lewisham Intensive Case

Management Scheme.' In S. Hunter (ed) *Dementia: Challenges and New Directions.* London: Jessica Kingsley Publishers.

Chamberlain, P. (1985) *Life Planning.* British Association of Behavioural Psychotherapy.

Chapman, A. and Marshall, M. (eds) (1993) *Dementia: New Skills for Social Workers.* London: Jessica Kingsley Publishers.

Chapman, K. and Oakes, P. (1995) 'Asking people with learning disabilities their view on direct psychological interventions.' *Clinical Psychology Forum,* No.81, July, 28–33.

Cheston, R. (1996) 'Stories and metaphors: Talking about the past in a psychotherapy group for people with dementia.' *Ageing and Society, 16,* 579–602.

Cheston, R. (1998) 'Psychotherapeutic work with people with dementia: A review of the literature.' *British Journal of Medical Psychology, 71,* 211–231.

Cheston, R. and Bender, M.P. (1999) 'Brains, minds and selves: Changing conceptions of the losses involved in dementia.' *British Journal of Medical Psychology, 72* (2) 203–216.

Cheston, R. and Peak, J. (1999) 'A single case investigation of the effects of Simulated Presence Therapy on people with dementia.' (forthcoming).

Church, M. and Wattis, J.P. (1988) 'Psychological approaches to the assessment and treatment of the elderly.' In J.P. Wattis and I. Hindmarch (eds) *Psychological Assessment of the Elderly.* Edinburgh: Churchill Livingstone.

Clarke, C.L. and Keady, J. (1996) 'Researching dementia care and family caregiving: Extending ethical responsibilities.' *Health Care in Later Life, 1,* 2, 87–95.

Clarke, M., Lowry, R. and Clarke, S. (1986) 'Cognitive impairment in the elderly – a community survey.' *Age & Ageing, 15,* 278–284.

Collins, H. and Pinch, T. (1993) *The Golem: What Everyone Should Know About Science.* Cambridge: Cambridge University Press.

Cohen, D., Kennedy, G. and Eisdorfer, C. (1984) 'Phases of change in the patient with Alzheimer's dementia.' *Journal of American Geriatric Society, 32,* 11–15.

Cooper, J.K., Mungas, D. and Weiler, P.G. (1990) 'Relation of cognitive status and abnormal behaviors in Alzheimer's disease.' *Journal of the American Geriatric Society, 38,* 867–870.

Cotrell, V. and Lein, L. (1993) 'Awareness and denial in the Alzheimer's disease victim.' *Journal of Gerontological Social Work, 19,* 3/4, 115–132.

Cotrell, V. and Schulz, R. (1993) 'The perspective of the patient with Alzheimer's disease: A neglected dimension of dementia research.' *Gerontologist, 33,* 2, 205–211.

Cottman, C. (1994) 'Report of Alzheimer's Disease working group A.' *Neurobiological Ageing, 15,* Supplement 2, S17–S22.

Couch, A. and Keniston, K. (1960) 'Yeasayers and Naysayers: Agreeing response set as a personality variable.' *Journal of Abnormal and Social Psychology, 60,* 151–174.

Coupland, J., Nussbaum, J.F. and Coupland, N. (1991) 'The reproduction of aging and ageism in intergenerational talk.' In N. Coupland, H. Giles and J.M. Wiemann (eds) *'Miscommunication' and Problematic Talk.* London: Sage.

Creutzfeldt, H.G. (1920) 'Uber eine eigenartige herdformige Erkrankungen der zentral nervensystem.' *Zeit Gesamte Neurol Psychiatrie, 57,* 1–18.

Crisp, J. (1995) 'Making sense of the stories that people with Alzheimer's tell: A journey with my mother.' *Nursing Inquiry, 2,* 133–140.

Cummings, J., Miller, B., Hill, M.A. (1987) 'Neuropsychiatric aspects of multi-infarct dementia and dementia of the Alzheimer type.' *Archives of Neurology, 44,* 389–393.

Cummings, J.L. and Victoroff, J.L. (1990) 'Noncognitive neuropsychiatric syndromes in Alzheimer's disease.' *Neuropsychiatry, Neuropsychology and Behavioral Neurology, 3,* 140–158.

Cupach, W.R. and Metts, S. (1994) *Facework.* London: Sage.

Dahlberg, C.C. and Jaffe, J. (1977) *Stroke: A Doctor's Personal Story of His Recovery.* New York: Norton.

Dant, T., Carley, M., Gearing, B. and Johnson, M. (1989) *Care for Elderly People at Home – A Research and Development Project in Collaboration with the Gloucester Health Authority: Final Report.* Milton Keynes: Department of Health and Social Welfare, Open University.

David, A.S. (1990) 'Insight and psychosis.' *British Journal of Psychiatry, 156,* 798–808.

David, P. (1991) 'Effectiveness of group work with the cognitively impaired older adult.' *Journal of Alzheimer's Care and Related Disorders and Research, 6,* 4, 10–16.

Davis, R. (1989) *My Journey into Alzheimer's Disease.* Amersham: Buckinghamshire: Scripture Press.

Department of Health (1990) *NHS and Community Care Act.* London: HMSO.

Department of Health (1995) *Carers (Recognition and Services) Act.* London: HMSO.

Department of Health (1996) *Carers (Recognition and Services) Act 1995: Practice Guidance.* London: HMSO.

Department of Health (1996a) *NHS Psychotherapy Services in England: Review of Strategic Policy.* London: NHS Executive.

Dick, L.P., Gallagher-Thompson, D. and Thompson, L.W. (1996) 'Cognitive behavioural therapy.' In R.T. Woods (ed) *Handbook of Clinical Psychology of Ageing.* Chichester: Wiley.

Downs, M., Carr, J., Chapman, A., Dunlop, A., Goldsmith, M., McLennan, J. and Murphy, C. (1994) *Dementia: A Literature Review for the Northern Ireland Dementia Policy Scrutiny.* University of Stirling: Dementia Services Development Centre.

Drayton, M. (1995) 'The emotional impact of schizophrenia.' *Clinical Psychology Forum, 28,* 15–20.

Duff, G. and Peach, E. (1994) *Mutual Support Groups: A Response to the Early and Often Forgotten Stage of Dementia.* Report, Dementia Services Development Centre, University of Stirling.

Edwards, A.L. (1957) *The Social Desirability Variable in Personality Research.* New York: Dryden Press.

Edwards, D., Potter, J. and Middleton, D. (1992) 'Towards a discursive psychology of remembering.' *The Psychologist, 5,* 10, 441–446.

Egan, G. (1994) *The Skilled Helper.* Pacific Grove, California: Brooks/Cole.

Ellis, A. (1962) *Reason and Emotion in Psychotherapy.* New York: Lyle Stuart.

Emerson, C. and Frampton, I. (1996) 'A psychological treatment approach to memory problems.' *Clinical Psychology Forum, 97,* November, 13–17.

Erikson, E.H. (1977) *Childhood and Society.* London: Granada.

Erikson, E.H. (1985) *The Life Cycle Completed*. New York: Norton.

Esquirol, J.E.D. (1838) *Des maladies mentales considerees sous les rapports medical, hygienique and medico-legal*. Two volumes. Paris.

Estes, C.L. and Binney, E.A. (1989) 'The biomedicalization of aging: Changes and dilemmas.' *Gerontologist, 29*, 587–596.

Feil, N. (1990) *Validation: The Feil Method*. Cleveland, Ohio: Edward Feil Productions. First published 1982.

Feil, N. (1992) 'Validation therapy.' In G. Jones and B. Miesen (eds) *Care-giving in Dementia*. London: Routledge.

Feil, N. (1993) *The Validation Breakthrough: Simple Techniques for Communicating with People with 'Alzheimer's-Type Dementia.'* Baltimore: Health Promotions Inc.

Fennell, G., Phillipson, C. and Evers, H. (1988) *The Sociology of Old Age*. Milton Keynes: Open University.

Fischer, O. (1907) 'Miliare nekrosen mit drusigen Wucherungen der Neurofibrillen, eine negelmässige Veränderung der Hirnrinde bei sender Demenz.' *Mschr. Psychiat. Neurol., 22*, 361–372.

Fish, F. (1968) *An Outline of Psychiatry for Students and Practitioners*. Bristol: John Wright.

Flynn, F.G., Cummings, J.L. and Gorbein, J. (1991) 'Delusions in dementia syndromes: Investigation of behavioural and neuropsychological correlates.' *Journal of Neuropsychology and Clinical Neuroscience, 3*, 364–370.

Folstein, M.F., Folstein, S.E. and McHugh, P.R. (1975) 'Mini-Mental State: A practical guide for grading the cognitive state of patients for the clinician.' *Journal of Psychiatric Research, 12*, 189–198.

Forster, M. (1989) *Have the Men had Enough?* London: Penguin.

Foucault, M. (1967) *Madness and Civilization*. London: Tavistock.

Fox, P. (1989) 'From senility to Alzheimer's Disease: The rise of the Alzheimer's Disease Movement.' *Millbank Quarterly, 67*, 1, 58–102.

Frank, B.A. (1955) 'People with dementia can communicate – if we are able to hear.' In T. Kitwood and S. Benson (eds) *The New Culture of Dementia Care*. London: Hawker.

Freud, S. (1953) 'On psychotherapy.' In *The Standard Edition of the Complete Psychological Works of Sigmund Freud*, Volume 7. London: Hogarth Press. First published 1905.

Freud, S. (1954) *The Interpretation of Dreams*. London: Allen and Unwin. 'Der Traumdeutung' first published Leipzig and Vienna by Franz Deuticke, 1900.

Freud, S. (1955) 'Introductory Lectures (1916–1917).' In J. Strachey (ed) *The Standard Edition of the Completed Psychological Works of Sigmund Freud*, Volume 16. London: Hogarth Press.

Freud, S. (1957) 'Mourning and Melancholia.' In J. Strachey (ed) *The Standard Edition of the Complete Psychological Works of Sigmund Freud*, Volume 14. London: Hogarth Press. First published in 1917.

Freud, S. (1958) 'Psycho-analytic notes on an autobiographical account of a case of paranoia (dementia paranoides).' In *The Standard Edition of the Complete Psychological Works*, Volume 12. London: Hogarth Press.

Freud, S. (1974) 'Indexes and Bibliographies.' In *The Standard Edition of the Complete Psychological Works*, Volume 24. London: Hogarth Press.

Froggatt, A. (1988) 'Self-awareness in early dementia.' In B. Gearing, M. Johnson and T. Heller (eds) *Mental Health Problems in Old Age: A Reader.* Milton Keynes: Open University Press.

Gatz, I. (1995) 'Early stage Alzheimer's patients find comfort in their own support group.' *Alzheimer's Disease International Global Perspective Newsletter 6,* 1, 6–7.

Gay, P. (1988) *Freud: A Life for Our Time.* London: Papermac.

Georgiades, N. and Phillimore, L. (1975) 'The myth of the hero-innovator and alternative strategies for organizational change.' In C. Kiernan and E. Woodford (eds) *Behaviour Modification with the Severely Retarded.* Amsterdam: Elsevier.

Giles, H. (1991) '"Gosh, you don't look it!": A sociolinguistic construction of ageing.' *The Psychologist, 3,* 99–106.

Gilewski, M.J. (1986) 'Group therapy with cognitively impaired older adults.' *Clinical Gerontology, 5,* 3–4, 281–296.

Gilleard, C.J. (1984) *Living with Dementia.* London: Croom Helm.

Gilleard, J. and Gwilliam, C. (1996) 'Sharing the diagnosis: A survey of memory disorders clinics: Their policies on informing people with dementia and their families, and the support they offer.' *International Journal of Geriatric Psychiatry, 11,* 11, 1001–1003.

Glaser, B.G. and Strauss, A.L. (1967) *The Discovery of Grounded Theory.* Chicago: Aldine.

Goffman, E. (1959) *The Presentation of Self in Everyday Life.* Doubleday, Anchor: New York.

Goffman, E. (1963) *Stigma.* Englewood Cliffs, New Jersey: Prentice Hall.

Goffman, E. (1967) *Interaction Ritual: Essays on Face-to-face Behaviour.* New York: Pantheon.

Goffman, E. (1991) *Asylums: Essays in the Social Situation of Mental Patients and Other Inmates.* Harmondsworth: Penguin.

Golden, R. (1995) 'Dementia and Alzheimer's Disease: Indications, diagnosis and treatment.' *Minn Med, 78,* 1, 25–29.

Golding, E. (1988) *MEAMS: The Middlesex Elderly Assessment of Mental State.* Bury St Edmunds, Suffolk: Thames Valley Test Co.

Goldsmith, M. (1996) *Hearing the Voice of People with Dementia.* London: Jessica Kingsley Publishers.

Gordon, D. and Spicker, P. (1997) 'Demography, needs and planning: The challenge of a changing population.' In S. Hunter (ed) *Dementia: Challenges and New Directions.* London: Jessica Kingsley Publishers.

Goudie, F. and Stokes, G. (1989) 'Dealing with confusion.' *Nursing Times,* September 20, 38.

Greene, J.A., Ingram, T.A. and Johnson, W. (1993) 'Group psychotherapy for patients with dementia.' *Southern Medical Journal, 86,* 9, 1033–1035.

Gubrium, J. (1986) *Oldtimer's and Alzheimer's: The Descriptive Organisation of Senility.* Greenwich Connecticut: Jai Press Inc.

Gubrium, J. (1987) 'Structuring and destructuring the course of illness: The Alzheimer's Disease experience.' *Sociology of Health and Illness, 9,* 1–24.

Gurland, B.J., Kuriansky, J.B., Sharpe, L., Simon, R., Stiller, P. and Birkett, P. (1977) 'The Comprehensive Assessment and Referral Evaluation (CARE) Rationale, development and reliability.' *International Journal of Ageing and Human Development,* 8, 9– 42.

Gurland, B., Copeland, J., Kuriansky, J., Kellerer, M., Sharpe, I. and Dean, L.L. (1983) *The Mind and Mood of Ageing: Mental Health Problems of the Community Elderly in New York and London.* London: Croom Helm.

Hachinski, V.C., Lassen, N.A. and Marshall, J. (1974) 'Multi-infarct dementia: A cause of mental deterioration in the elderly.' *Lancet, ii,* 207–210.

Hachinski, V.C., Iliff, L.D., Zihka, E., Duboulay, G.H., McAllister, V.L., Marshall, J., Russell, R.W.R. and Symon, L. (1975) 'Cerebral blood flow in dementia.' *Archives of Neurology, 32,* 632–637.

Haggerty, A.D. (1990) 'Psychotherapy for patients with Alzheimer's Disease.' *Advances, 7,* 1, 55–60.

Hagnell, O., Ojesso, L. and Rorsman, B. (1992) 'Incidence of dementia in the Lundby study.' *Neuroepidemiology 1* (suppl. 1), 61–66.

Hall, G.R. and Buckwalter, K.C. (1987) 'Progressively lowered stress threshold: A conceptual model for care of adults with Alzheimer's Disease.' *Archives of Psychiatric Nursing, 1,* 6, 399–406.

Hamilton, E. (1978) *Fish's Outline of Psychiatry,* 3rd edition. Bristol: Wright.

Hamilton, H.E. (1994) *Conversations with an Alzheimer's Patient.* Cambridge: Cambridge University Press.

Handel, G. (ed) (1968) *The Psychosocial Interior of the Family.* London: Allen and Unwin.

Harding, N. and Palfry, C. (1997) *The Social Construction of Dementia.* London: Jessica Kingsley Publishers.

Harms, E. (1971) 'Introduction.' In E. Kraepelin *Dementia Praecox and Paraphrenia.* Huntington, New York: Robert E. Krieger.

Harper, D.J. (1992) 'Defining delusion and the serving of professional interests: The case of "paranoia".' *British Journal of Medical Psychology, 65,* 357–369.

Harper, D.J. (1994) 'The professional construction of "paranoia" and the discursive use of diagnostic criteria.' *British Journal of Medical Psychology, 67,* 131–143.

Hart, S. and Semple, J.M. (1994) *Neuropsychology and the Dementias.* Hove, Sussex: Lawrence Erlbaum.

Hausman, C. (1992) 'Dynamic psychotherapy with elderly demented patients.' In G.M.M. Jones and B.M.L. Miesen (eds) *Care-giving in Dementia.* London: Tavistock/Routledge.

Hazell, J., Driver, H. and Shalan, D. (1996) 'Obtaining service criticism from older adults.' *PSIGE Newsletter,* No.57.

Health Advisory Service (1982) *The Rising Tide: Developing Services for Mental Illness in Old Age.* Sutherland House, Sutton, Surrey, SH2 5AN.

Healy, D. (1997) *Psychiatric Drugs Explained* (2nd edition). London: Mosby.

Heider, F. (1958) *The Psychology of Interpersonal Relations.* New York: Wiley.

Henderson, A.S. (1983) 'The coming epidemic of dementia.' *Australian and New Zealand Journal of Psychiatry, 17,* 117–127.

Hendrie, H.C.; Osuntokun, B.O.; Hall, K.S. *et al.* (1995) 'Prevalence of Alzheimer's disease and dementia in two communities: Nigerian Africans and African Americans.' *American Journal of Psychiatry, 152,* 1485–1492.

Heywood, B. (1994) *Caring for Maria.* Shaftesbury, Dorset: Element.

Hildebrand, P. (1986) 'Dynamic psychotherapy with the elderly.' In I. Hanley and M. Gilhooly (eds) *Psychological Therapies for the Elderly*. London: Croom Helm

Hill, K.; O'Brien, J.; Morant, N.J. and Levy, R. (1995) 'User expectations of a memory clinic.' *Clinical Psychology Forum, 10,* 9–11.

Hockey, J. and James, A. (1993) *Growing Up and Growing Old: Ageing and Dependency in the Life Course*. London: Sage.

Hoff, P. (1991) 'Alzheimer and his time.' In G.E. Berrios and H.L. Freeman (eds) *Alzheimer and the Dementias*. London: Royal Society of Medicine Services, 29–56.

Hofman, A. *et al.* (1991) 'The prevalence of dementia in Europe: A collaborative study of 1980–1990 findings.' *International Journal of Epidemiology, 20,* 736–748.

Holden, U. (1995) *Ageing, Neuropsychology and the 'New' Dementias*. London: Chapman and Hall.

Holden, U.P. and Woods, R.T. (1995) *Positive Approaches to Dementia Care* (3rd edition). Edinburgh: Churchill Livingstone.

Hollingshead, A.B. and Redlich, F.C. (1958) *Social Class and Mental Illness*. New York: Wiley.

Holmes, J. (1993) *John Bowlby and Attachment Theory*. London: Routledge.

Holmes, T.H. and Rahe, R.H. (1967) 'The social readjustment rating scale.' *Journal of Psychosomatic Research, 11,* 213–218.

Hunt, L., Marshall, M. and Rowlings, C. (eds) (1997) *Past Trauma in Late Life*. London: Jessica Kingsley Publishers.

Hunter, S. (ed) (1997) *Dementia: Challenges and New Directions*. London: Jessica Kingsley Publishers.

Ignatieff, M. (1993) *Scar Tissue*. London: Vintage Books.

Ikeda, M.; Mori, E.; Hirono, N.; Imamura, T.; Shimomura, T.; Ikejiri, Y. and Yamashita, H. (1998) 'Amnestic people with Alzheimer's disease who remember the Kobe earthquake.' *British Journal of Psychiatry, 172,* 425–428.

Illich, I. (1975) *Medical Nemesis: The Expropriation of Health*. London: Calder & Boyars.

Ineichen, B. (1987) 'Measuring the rising tide: How many dementia cases will there be by 2001?' *British Journal of Psychiatry, 150,* 193–200.

Ineichen, B. (1997) 'The prevalence of dementia and cognitive impairment in China.' *International Journal of Geriatric Psychiatry, 11,* 695–697.

Jackson, D. and Wonson, S. (1987) 'Alzheimer's re-socialization: A group approach towards improved social awareness among Alzheimer's patients.' *American Journal of Alzheimer's Care and Related Disorders and Research, 2,* 5, 31–35.

Jakob, A. (1921) 'Uber eine multiplen sklerose klinisch nahestehende erkrankung des zentralnerven system (spastiche Pseudosklerose) mit bemerkenswertem anatomischem befunde. Mitteilung eines vierten fallen.' *Med Klin, 17,* 372–376.

Jarvis, K. (1997) 'I remember me.' *Signpost 2,* 3, September.

Jenkins, R. and Phillips, G. (1996) *Giving a diagnosis of dementia: What is said, to whom?* Paper presented at PSIGE annual conference, Cardiff.

Johnson, M.; Gearing, B.; Dant, T. and Carley, M. (1989) *Care for Elderly People at Home: Final Report*. The Open University Dept. of Health and Social Welfare and Policy Studies Institute, Milton Keynes, Bucks.

Jones, E. (1964) *The Life and Work of Sigmund Freud*. Harmondsworth, Middlesex: Penguin.

Jones, S.N. (1995) 'An interpersonal approach to psychotherapy with older persons with dementia.' *Professional Psychology: Research and Practice, 26*, 6, 602–607.

Jung, C.G. (1933) *Modern Man in Search of a Soul.* New York: Harcourt.

Jung, G.G. (1938) *Psychology and Religion.* New Haven: Yale University Press.

Kahn, R.S. (1965) 'Comments.' In *Proceedings of the York House Institute on the Mentally Impaired Aged.* Philadelphia: Philadelphia Geriatric Centre.

Kaplan, E.S. (1990) 'Facing the loss of what makes us uniquely human: working with dementia patients.' In B. Genevay and R. Katz (eds) *Countertransference and Older Adults.* California: Sage.

Karlsson, T.; Bäckman, L.; Herlitz, A.; Nilsson, L.G.; Winblad, B. and Österlind, P.O. (1989) 'Memory improvement at different stages of Alzheimer's disease.' *Neuropsychologia, 27*, 5, 737–742.

Karpman, S. (1968) 'Fairy tales and script drama analysis.' *Transactional Analysis Bulletin, 7*, 39–43.

Katzman, R. and Karasu, T. (1975) 'Differential diagnosis of dementia.' In W. Fields (ed) *Neurological and Sensory Disorders in the Elderly.* New York: Stratton.

Kavanagh, S.; Schneider, J.; Knapp, M.; Neecham, J. and Netten, A. (1993) 'Elderly people with cognitive impairment: Costing possible changes in the balance of care.' *Health and Social Care, 1*, 69–80.

Kay, D.W.K. and Bergmann, K. (1980) 'Epidemiology of mental disorders among the aged in the community.' In J.E. Birren and R.B. Sloane (eds) *Handbook of Mental Health and Ageing.* Englewood Cliffs, New Jersey: Prentice Hall.

Keady, J. (1996) 'The experience of dementia: A review of the literature and implications for nursing practice.' *Journal of Clinical Nursing, 5*, 275–288.

Keady, J. (1997) 'Maintaining involvement: A meta-concept to describe the dynamics of dementia.' In M. Marshall (ed) *State of the Art in Dementia Care.* London: Centre for Policy on Ageing.

Keady, J. and Bender, M.P. (1998) 'Changing faces: The purpose and practice of assessing older adults with cognitive impairment.' *Health Care in Later Life, 3*, 2, 129–144.

Keady, J. and Nolan, M. (1994) 'Younger onset dementia: Developing a longitudinal model as a basis for a research agenda and as a guide to interventions with sufferers and carers.' *Journal of Advanced Nursing, 19*, 659–669.

Keady, J. and Nolan, M. (1995a) 'A stitch in time – Facilitating proactive interventions with dementia caregivers: The role of community practitioners.' *Journal of Psychiatric and Mental Health Nursing, 2*, 33–40.

Keady, J. and Nolan, M.R. (1995b) 'IMMEL: Assessing coping responses in the early stages of dementia.' *British Journal of Nursing, 4*, 309–314.

Keady, J. and Nolan, M.R. (1995c) 'IMMEL 2: Working to augment coping responses in early dementia.' *British Journal of Nursing, 4*, 377–380.

Keady, J., Nolan, M. and Gilliard, J. (1995) 'Listen to the voices of experience.' *Journal of Dementia Care, 3*, 3, 15–17.

Kempenaar, L. and McNamara, C. (1998) *Specific Sensory Stimulation: An Approach to Sensory Therapy for Carers.* Ayshire and Arran Community Health Care NHS Trust.

Kendrick, D.C. (1985) *The Kendrick Cognitive Tests for the Elderly.* Windsor, Berks: NFER-Nelson.

Kesey, K. (1973) *One Flew Over the Cuckoo's Nest.* London: Pan.

Khachaturian, Z.S. (1985) 'Diagnosis of Alzheimer's Disease.' *Archive of Neurology, 42,* 1097–1105.

Kierkegaard, S. (1954) *Fear and Trembling/The Sickness unto Death.* New York: Doubleday Anchor.

Killick, J. (1997) *You Are Words: Dementia Poems.* London: Hawker.

King's Fund (1986) *Living Well into Old Age.* A King's Fund project paper: London.

Kirk, S.A. and Kutchins, H. (1992) *The Selling of DSM: The Rhetoric of Science in Psychiatry.* New York: Aldine De Gruyter.

Kitwood, T. (1987) 'Dementia and its pathology: In brain, mind or society?' *Free Associations, 8,* 81–93.

Kitwood, T. (1988) 'The technical, the personal and the framing of dementia.' *Social Behaviour, 3,* 161–179.

Kitwood, T. (1990a) 'The dialectics of dementia: With particular reference to Alzheimer's Disease.' *Ageing and Society, 10,* 177–196.

Kitwood, T. (1990b) 'Psychotherapy and dementia.' *Newsletter of the Psychotherapy Section of the British Psychological Society, 8,* 40–56.

Kitwood, T. (1993) 'Person and process in dementia.' *International Journal of Geriatric Psychiatry, 8,* 541–545.

Kitwood, T. (1994) 'The concept of personhood and its implications for the care of those who have dementia.' *Caregiving in Dementia, 2.*

Kitwood, T. (1996) 'Positive long-term changes in dementia: Some preliminary observations.' *Journal of Mental Health, 4,* 133–144.

Kitwood, T. (1997a) 'The experience of dementia.' *Ageing and Mental Health, 1,* 1, 13–22.

Kitwood, T. (1997b) *Dementia Reconsidered: The Person Comes First.* Buckingham: Open University Press.

Kitwood, T. (undated) *Some Problematical Aspects of Dementia.* Bradford Dementia Research Group: unpublished.

Kitwood, T. and Benson, S. (eds) (1995) *The New Culture of Dementia Care.* London: Hawker Publications.

Kitwood, T. and Bredin, K. (1992) 'Toward a theory of dementia care: Personhood and well-being.' *Ageing and Society, 12,* 269–287.

Kitwood, T. and Bredin, K. (1994) *Evaluating Dementia Care: The Dementia Care Mapping Method.* Bradford University Dementia Group (sixth edition).

Klerman, G.L. (1984) 'The advantages of DSM-III.' *American Journal of Psychiatry, 141,* 539–542.

Knight, B. (1986) *Psychotherapy with the Older Adult.* Beverley Hills: Sage.

Knight, B. (1992) *Older Adults in Psychotherapy.* Newbury Park: Sage.

Knight, B.G.; Lutzky, S.M. and Macofsky-Urban, F. (1993) 'A meta-analytic review of interventions for caregiver distress: Recommendations for future research.' *Gerontologist, 33,* 2, 240–248.

Kraepelin, E. (1910) *Psychiatrie: Ein Lehrbuch fur Studierende und Arzte* (8th edition). Leipzig: Barth.

Kraepelin, E. (1919) *Dementia Praecox and Paraphrenia*: Translated by R.M. Barclay. Edinburgh: Livingstone.

Kraepelin, E. (1917) *One Hundred Years of Psychiatry*. London: Peter Owen.

Kraepelin, E. (1987) *Memoirs*. New York: Springer.

Kral, V. (1983) 'The relationship between senile dementia (Alzheimer type) and depression.' *Canadian Journal of Psychiatry, 28*, 304 –6.

Krebs-Roubicek, E.M. (1989) 'Group therapy with demented elderly.' *Alzheimer's Disease and Related Disorders*, 1261–1272.

Kübler-Ross, E. (1970) *On Death and Dying*. London: Tavistock.

Kuhlman, G.J.; Wilson, H.S.; Hutchinson, S.A. and Wallhagen, M. (1991) 'Alzheimer's disease and family caregiving: Critical synthesis of the literature and research agenda.' *Nursing Research, 40*, 6, 331–337.

Kuhn, T.S. (1962) *The Structure of Scientific Revolutions*. Chicago: University of Chicago.

LaBarge, E. and Trtanj, F. (1995) 'A support group for people in the early stages of dementia of the Alzheimer's type.' *Journal of Applied Gerontology, 14*, 3, 289–301.

Lachs, M.S.; Becker, J.T.; Siegal, A.P.; Miller, R.L. and Tinetti, M.E. (1992) 'Delusions and behavioural disturbance in cognitively impaired elderly persons.' *Journal of the American Geriatric Society, 40*, 8, 768–773.

Laing, R.D. (1959) *The Divided Self*. London: Tavistock.

Laing, R.D. (1967) *The Politics of Experience* and *The Bird of Paradise*. Harmondsworth Middlesex: Penguin.

Lawton, M.P. (1980a) *Environment and Ageing*. Los Angeles: Brooks/Cole.

Lawton, M.P. (1980b) 'Psychosocial and environmental approaches to the care of senile dementia patients.' In J.O. Cole and J.E. Barrett (eds) *Psychopathology in the Aged*. New York: Raven Press.

Lawton, M.P. and Brody, E. (1969) 'Assessment of older people: Self-maintaining and instrumental activities of daily living.' *Gerontologist, 9*, 179–186.

LeGoues, G. (1988) 'Le solutien de l'apperail psychique du dément.' *Psychologie Médicale, 20*, 7, 948–950.

Levin, E.; Sinclair, I. and Gorbach, P. (1983) *The Supporters of Confused Elderly Persons at Home, Vol. 3: Appendices*. London: National Institute of Social Work.

Levin, E.; Sinclair, I. and Gorbach, P. (1989) *Families, Services and Confusion in Old Age*. Aldershot: Avebury.

Levy, B. and Langer, E. (1994) 'Aging free from negative stereotypes: Successful memory in China and among the American deaf.' *Journal of Personality and Social Psychology, 66*, 6, 989–997.

Lewis, I.M. (1971) *Ecstatic Religion*. Harmondsworth, Middlesex: Penguin.

Ley, P. (1982) 'Giving information to patients.' In J.R. Eiser (ed) *Social Psychology and Behavioural Medicine*. London: Wiley.

Lindesay, J.; Briggs, K. and Murphy, E. (1989) 'The Guy's/Age Concern Survey: Prevalence rates of cognitive impairment, depression and anxiety in an urban elderly community.' *British Journal of Psychiatry, 155*, 317–329.

Lishman, W.A. (1987) *Organic Psychiatry* (2nd edition). Blackwell: Oxford.

Littlewood, R. and Lipsedge, M. (1989) *Aliens and Alienists* (2nd edition). London: Unwin Hyman.

Mace, C. and Margison, F. (1997) 'Attachment and psychotherapy – an overview.' *British Journal of Medical Psychology, 70,* 209–215.

McCullough, D.R. (1980) *The Needs of Carers of Elderly People with Dementia.* Glasgow: Strathclyde Regional Council.

McGowin, D.F. (1993) *Living in the Labyrinth: A Personal Journey Through the Maze of Alzheimer's Disease.* Cambridge: Mainsail Press.

McGrath, A.M. and Jackson, G.A. (1996) 'Survey of neuroleptic prescribing in residents of nursing homes in Glasgow.' *British Medical Journal, 312,* 9th March, 611–612.

McHenry, L.C. (1969) *Garrison's History of Neurology.* Springfield, Illinois: Thomas.

McMenemey, W.H. (1970) 'Alois Alzheimer and his disease.' In G.E.W. Wolstenholme and M. O'Connor (eds) *Alzheimer's Disease and Related Conditions.* London: Churchill.

McNamee, S. and Gergen, K.S. (eds) (1992) *Therapy as Social Construction.* London: Sage.

McPherson, F.M. and Tregaskis, D. (1985) 'The short-term stability of the survey version of CAPE.' *British Journal of Clinical Psychology, 24,* 205–206.

McShane, R.; Keene, J.; Gedling, K.; Fairburn, C.; Jacoby, R. and Hope, T. (1997) 'Do neuroleptic drugs hasten cognitive decline in dementia? Prospective study with necroscopy follow-up.' *British Medical Journal, 314,* 266–270.

Maguire, C.P.; Kirby, M.; Coen, R.; Coakley, D.; Lawlor, B.A. and O'Neill, D. (1996) 'Family members' attitudes toward telling the patient with Alzheimer's disease their diagnosis.' *British Medical Journal, 313,* 529–530.

Maher, B.A. (1970) *Principles of Psychopathology.* New York: McGraw-Hill.

Maher, B.A. (1973) *Contemporary Abnormal Psychology.* Harmondsworth: Penguin.

Mahl, G.F. and Schulze, G. (1964) 'Psychological research in the extra-linguistic area.' In T. Sebeok, A.S. Hayes and M.C. Bateson (eds) *Approaches to Semiotics.* London: Mouton.

Main, M. (1996) 'Introduction to the special section on attachment and Psychopathology: 2. Overview of the field of attachment.' *Journal of Consulting and Clinical Psychology, 64,* 2, 237–243.

Maisondieu, J. (1995) 'La Psychothérapie du Dément: Un Psychothérapie au Point Mort Faute de Demande?' *Psychologie Médicale, 27,* 3, 132–135.

Markova, I. and Berrios, G.E. (1995) 'Insight in clinical psychiatry.' *Journal of Nervous and Mental Disease, 183,* 12, 743–751.

Marshall, M. (1996) *I Can't Place This Place At All: Working with People with Dementia and their Carers.* Birmingham: Venture.

Marshall, M. (1998) 'How it helps to see dementia as a disability.' *Journal of Dementia Care,* January/February, 15–17.

Masson, J. M. (1985) *The Assault on Truth.* Harmondsworth, Middlesex: Penguin.

Maurer, K.; Volk, S. and Gerbaldo, H. (1997) 'Auguste D and Alzheimer's disease.' *Lancet, 349* (no. 9064), 1546–1549.

Maxim, J. and Bryan, K. (1994) *Language of the Elderly.* London: Whurr.

Maxmen, J. (1985) *The New Psychiatrists.* New York: New American Library.

Melzer, D. (1998) 'New drug treatment for Alzheimer's disease: Lessons for healthcare policy.' *British Medical Journal, 316*, 16, 7 March, 762–764.

Middleton, D. and Edwards, D. (1990) *Collective Remembering.* London: Sage.

Miesen, B. (1992) 'Attachment theory and dementia.' In G. Jones and B.M.L. Miesen (eds) *Care Giving in Dementia: Research and Applications.* London: Routledge.

Miesen, B. (1993) 'Alzheimer's disease, the phenomenon of parent fixation and Bowlby's attachment theory.' *International Journal of Geriatric Psychiatry, 8,* 147–153.

Miesen, B. (1995) *Psychic Pain Surfacing in Dementia: From New to Old Sore?* Paper given at the European colloquium in Therapeutic work with older people, Stirling, June.

Miesen, B. and Jones, G.T.Y. (1997) 'Psychic pain resurfacing in dementia: from new to past trauma?' In L. Hunt, M. Marshall and C. Rawlings (eds) *Past Trauma in Late Life: European Perspectives on Therapeutic Work with Older People.* London: Jessica Kingsley Publishers.

Miller, A.D. (1989) 'Opportunities for psychotherapy in the management of dementia.' *Journal of Geriatric Psychiatry and Neurology, 2,* Jan–March, 11–17.

Miller, E. (1977) *Abnormal Ageing: The Psychology of Senile and Presenile Dementia.* London: Wiley.

Miller, E. and Hague, F. (1975) 'Some characteristics of verbal behaviour in pre-senile dementia.' *Psychological Medicine, 5,* 255–259.

Miller, E. and Morris, R. (1993) *The Psychology of Dementia.* Chichester, John Wiley.

Miller, E.J. and Gwynne, G. (1972) *Life Apart: A Pilot Study of Residential Institutions for the Physically Handicapped and the Young Chronic Sick.* London: Tavistock.

Mills, M.A. (1997) 'Narrative, identity and dementia: a study of emotion and narrative in older people with dementia.' *Ageing and Society, 17,* 673–698.

Mills, M.A. and Walker, J.M. (1994) 'Memory, mood and dementia: A case study.' *Journal of Ageing Studies, 8,* 1, 17–27.

Mills, M.A.; Coleman, P.; Jerrome, D.; Conroy, C. and Meade, R. (1998) 'Changing patterns of dementia care: The influence of attachment theory in staff training.' *British Journal of Social Work,* in press.

Mischel, W. (1968) *Personality and Assessment.* New York: Wiley.

Moniz-Cook, E. and Woods, R.T (1997) 'The role of memory clinics and psychosocial intervention in the early stages of dementia.' *International Journal of Geriatric Psychiatry, 12,* 1143–1145.

Morel, B.A. (1852) *Etudes Cliniques sur les Maladies Mentales.* Paris: Masson.

Morgan, K.; Lilley, J.; Arie, T.; Byrne, J.; Jones, R. and Waite, J. (1992) 'Incidence of dementia: Preliminary findings from the Nottingham longitudinal study of activity and ageing.' *Neuroepidemiology, 1* (suppl. 1), 80–83.

Moritz, D.J. and Petitti, D.B. (1993) 'Association of education with reported age of onset and severity of Alzheimer's disease at presentation: Implications for the use of clinical samples.' *American Journal of Epidemiology, 137,* 4, 456–462.

Morris, R.G.; Morris, L.W. and Britton, P.G. (1988) 'Factors affecting the emotional well-being of the caregivers of dementia sufferers.' *British Journal of Psychiatry, 153,* 147–156.

Morrow, S.L.; Allen, S.C. and Campbell, B.W. (1997) 'Enhancing quality of life in AIDS-related dementia.' *Psychotherapy, 34,* 3, 324–332.

Mortel, K.F.; Meyer, J.S.; Herod, B. and Thornby, J. (1994/1995) 'Education and occupation as risk factors for dementias of the Alzheimer's and Ischemic Vascular types.' *Dementia, 6*, 1, 55–62.

Mortimer, J.A. and Graves, A.B. (1993) 'Education and other socioeconomic determinants of dementia and Alzheimer's disease.' *Neurology, 43*, 8, S4, S39–S44.

Morton, I. (1997) 'Beyond validation.' In I. Norman and S. Redfern (eds) *Mental Health Care for Elderly People*. Edinburgh: Churchill Livingstone.

Morton, I. and Bleathman, C. (1988) 'Does it matter whether it's Tuesday or Friday?' *Nursing Times, 84*, 6, February 10, 25–28.

Mowle-Clark, K.; Bender, M. and Brown, K. (1992) 'Discovering the magic circle.' *Therapy Weekly*, December 3, 8.

Moyes, M. and Christie, H. (1998a) 'Focus on each individual's experience and emotions.' *Journal of Dementia Care, 6*, 4, July/August, 16–18.

Moyes, M. and Christie, H. (1998b) 'Structuring groups to make psychotherapy possible.' *Journal of Dementia Care, 6*, 5, 15–17.

Murphy, E. (1982) 'Social origins of depression in old age.' *British Journal of Psychiatry, 141*, 135–142.

Murphy, E. (ed) (1986) *Affective Disorders in the Elderly*. Edinburgh: Churchill Livingstone.

Murphy, E. (1986) 'Social factors in depression.' In E. Murphy (ed) *Affective Disorders in the Elderly*. Edinburgh: Churchill Livingstone.

Murray, A. (1996) 'Listening to people with dementia.' *Signpost, 1*, 35, 13–14.

Myers-Arràzola, L. and Bizzini, L. (1995) 'Psychothérapie Cognitive et Patients Atteints de Démence Débutante.' *Psychologie Médicale, 27*, 3, 178–179.

Nelson, H.E. (1991) *National Adult Reading Test* (N.A.R.T.) Test Manual: 2nd edition. Windsor, Berks: NFER-NELSON.

Nelson-Jones, R. (1990) *Human Relationship Skills*, 2nd edition. London: Cassell.

Norman, A. (1985) *Triple Jeopardy: Growing Old in a Second Homeland*. London: Centre for Policy on Ageing.

Norris, A.D. (1986) *Reminiscence with Older People*. Bicester, Oxon: Winslow.

Norris, A.D. and Abu el Eileh, N. (1982) 'Reminiscing – a therapy for both elderly patients and their staff.' *Nursing Times, 78*, 32, 1368–1369.

Oakley, D.P. (1965) 'Senile dementia: Some aetiological factors.' *British Journal of Psychiatry, 111*, 414–419.

O'Connor, D. (1993) 'The impact of dementia: A self psychological perspective.' *Journal of Gerontological Social Work, 20*, 3/4, 113–128.

O'Connor, D.W.; Pollitt, P.A.; Brook, C.D.P.; Reiss, B.B. and Roth, M. (1991) 'Does early intervention reduce the number of elderly people with dementia admitted to institutions for long term care?' *British Medical Journal, 302*, 871–875.

Orrell, M. and Bebbington, P. (1995) 'Life events and senile dementia.' *British Journal of Psychiatry, 166*, 613–620.

Orrell, M. and Woods, R. (1996) 'Tacrine and psychological therapies in dementia – no contest?' *International Journal of Geriatric Psychiatry, 11*, 189–192.

Orrell, M.W. and Davies, A.D.M. (1994) 'Life events in the elderly.' *International Review of Psychiatry, 6*, 59–71.

Osgood, C.E.; Suci, G.J. and Tannenbaum, P.H. (1957) *The Measurement of Meaning.* Urbana, Illinois: University of Illinois.

Osuntokun, B.O. *et al.* (1992) 'Cross-cultural studies in Alzheimer's disease.' *Ethnic Dis, 2,* 352–357.

Ott, A.; Breteler, M.M.B.; Vanharskamp, F.; Claus, J.J.; Vandercammen, T.J.M.; Grobbee, D.E. and Hofman, A. (1995) 'Prevalence of Alzheimer's-disease and vascular dementia – association with education: the Rotterdam Study.' *British Medical Journal, 310* (1985), 970–973.

Parker, G. (1997) 'Coping with caring for a person with dementia.' In S. Hunter (ed) *Dementia: Challenges and New Directions.* London: Jessica Kingsley Publishers.

Parkes, C.M. (1971) 'Psycho-social transitions: A field for study.' *Social Science and Medicine, 5,* 101–115.

Parkes, C.M. (1975) 'What becomes of redundant world models? A contribution to the study of adaptation to change.' *British Journal of Medical Psychology, 48,* 131–137.

Parkes, C.M. (1986) *Bereavement* (2nd edition). Harmondsworth, Middlesex: Penguin.

Paterson, D. (1980) 'Is your brain really necessary?' *World Medicine,* May 3, 21–24.

Pattie, A.H. and Gilleard, C.J. (1976) 'The Clifton assessment schedule – further validation of a psychogeriatric assessment schedule.' *British Journal of Psychiatry, 129,* 68–72.

Pattie, A.H. and Gilleard, C.J. (1979) *Manual for the Clifton Assessment Procedures for the Elderly (CAPE).* Sevenoaks, Kent: Hodder and Stoughton.

Peach, E. and Duff, G. (1991) 'Mutual support groups: A response to the early and often forgotten stage of dementia.' *Practice, 6,* 2, 147–157.

Peak, J. (1999) 'An evaluation of simulated presence therapy in terms of attachment theory and the experience of dementia.' Dissertation submitted for BSc in Psychology with Sociology, University of Bath.

Perusini, G. (1909) 'Uber Klinisch und histologisch eigenartige psychische Erkrankungen des späteren Lebensalters.' In F. Nissl and A. Alzheimer (eds) *Histologische und Histopathologische Arbeiten.* Jena: Verlag G. Fischer, 297–351.

Perusini, G. (1911) 'Sul valore nosografico di alcuni reperti istopatologici: Caratteristiche per la senilità.' *Rivista Italiana di Neuropatologia Psichiatria ed Elettroterapia, 4,* 193–213.

Pick, A. (1906) 'Uber einen weiterer symptomkomplex in Rahmen der Dementia senilis, bedingt durch umschriebene starkere Hirnatrophie (gemische Apraxie).' *Monatschrift für Psychiatrie und Neurologie, 19,* 97–108.

Ploton, L. (1995) 'Hypothèses de la persistance d'un appareil rélationnel pertinent chez les déments séniles.' *Psychologie Médicale, 27,* 3, 156–159.

Podoll, K.; Vonderstein, B.; Stuhlmann, W. and Kretschmar, C. (1992) 'Transitional objects as regression phenomena in demented patients.' *Nervenarzt, 63,* 5, 276–280.

Pollitt, P.A. (1997) 'The problem of dementia in Australian Aboriginal and Torres Strait Islander communities: An overview.' *International Journal of Geriatric Psychiatry, 12,* 155–163.

Powell, Proctor, L. and Miller, E. (1982) 'Reality Orientation: A critical appraisal.' *British Journal of Psychiatry, 140,* 457–463.

Pritchard, J.C. (1842) *On the Different Forms of Insanity in Relation to Jurisprudence.* London.

Rabbitt, P. (1996) 'Speed of processing and ageing.' In R.T. Woods (ed) *Handbook of the Clinical Psychology of Ageing.* Chichester: Wiley, 59–72.

Reding, M.; Haycox, J. and Blass, J. (1985) 'Depression in patients referred to a dementia clinic.' *Archives of Neurology, 42,* 894–896.

Reisberg, B.; Ferris, S.M., de Leon, M. and Crook, T. (1982) 'The Global Deterioration Scale for assessment of primary degenerative dementia.' *American Journal of Psychiatry, 139,* 1136–1139.

Rice, K. and Warner, N. (1994) 'Breaking the bad news: What do psychiatrists tell patients with dementia about their illness?' *International Journal of Geriatric Psychiatry, 9,* 467–471.

Richards, M. (1997) 'Cross-cultural studies of dementia.' In C. Holmes and R. Howard (eds) *Advances in Old Age Psychiatry: Chromosomes to Community Care.* Petersfield, UK: Wrightson Biomedical.

Richardson, E.P. (1977) 'Introduction.' In D.A. Rottenberg and F.H. Hochberg (eds) *Neurological Classics in Modern Translation.* New York: Hafner Press.

Ripich, D.N.; Vertes, D.; Whitehouse, P.; Fulton, S. and Ekelman, B. (1991) 'Turn-taking and speech act patterns in the discourse of senile dementia of the Alzheimer's type patients.' *Brain and Language, 40,* 330–343.

Roach, M. (1985) *Another Name for Madness.* Borton: Houghton Mifflon.

Robinson, B. (1995) 'Death of destruction of will – lest we forget.' *Archives of Internal Medicine, 155,* 20, 2250–2251.

Rodin, J. and Langer, E. (1980) 'Aging labels: The decline of control and the fall of self-esteem.' *Journal of Social Issues, 36,* 2, 12–29.

Rogers, C.R. (1961) *On Becoming a Person: A Therapist's View of Psychotherapy.* Boston: Houghton Mifflin.

Rogers, C.R. (1978) *Carl Rogers on Personal Power.* London: Constable.

Rogers, C.R. and Stevens, B. (1971) *Person to Person: The Problem of Being Human.* New York: Pocket Books.

Rosen, G. (1968) *Madness in Society.* Chicago: University of Chicago Press.

Roth, M.; Huppert, F.A.; Tyn, E. and Mountjoy, C.Q. (1988) *The Cambridge Examination for Mental Disorders in the Elderly.* Cambridge: Cambridge University Press.

Roth, M.; Tomlinson, B.E. and Blessed, G. (1966) 'Correlations between scores for dementia and counts of senile plaques in cerebral grey matter of elderly subjects.' *Nature, 209,* 109–110.

Roth, M.; Tomlinson, B.E. and Blessed, G. (1967) 'The relationship between quantative measures of dementia and of degenerative changes in the cerebral grey matter of elderly subjects.' *Proc. R. Soc., Med., 60,* 254–260.

Roth, M.; Tyn, E.; Mountjoy, C.Q.; Huppert, F.A.; Hendrie, H.; Verma, S. and Goddard, R. (1986) 'CAMDEX: a standardised instrument for the diagnosis of mental disorder in the elderly with special reference to the early detection of dementia.' *British Journal of Psychiatry, 149,* 698–709.

Rothschild, D. (1937) 'Pathologic changes in senile psychoses and their psychobiologic significance.' *American Journal of Psychiatry, 93,* 757–788.

Rothschild, D. (1942) 'Neuropathologic changes in arteriosclerotic psychoses and their psychiatric significance.' *Archives of Neurology and Psychiatry, 48,* 417–436.

Rothschild, D. and Sharp, M.L. (1941) 'The origin of senile psychoses: Neuropathologic factors and factors of a more personal nature.' *Diseases of the Nervous System, 2,* 49–54.

Rowe, D. (1994) *Time on Our Side: Growing in Wisdom, Not Growing Old.* London: Harper Collins.

Rutter, M. (1995) 'Clinical Implications of attachment concepts: Retrospect and prospect.' *Journal of Child Psychology and Psychiatry, 36,* 4, 549–571.

Ryden, M. (1988) 'Aggressive behaviour in persons with dementia who live in the community.' *Alzheimer's Disease and Associated Disorders, 2,* 342–355.

Sabat, S.R. (1994) 'Excess disability and malignant social psychology: A case study of Alzheimer's disease.' *Journal of Community and Applied Social Psychology, 4,* 157–166.

Sabat, S.R. and Harré, R. (1992) 'The construction and deconstruction of self in Alzheimer's disease.' *Ageing and Society, 12,* 443–461.

Sabat, S.R.; Fath, H.; Moghaddam, F.M. and Harré, R. (1999) 'The termination of self and the loss of self-esteem: Lessons from the culture of AD sufferers.' *Culture and Society,* in press.

Sabsay, S. and Platt, M. (1985) 'Weaving the cloak of competence.' Chapter 5 in S. Sabsay and M. Platt (eds) *Social Settings, Stigma and Communication Competence.* Amsterdam: Benjamin.

Sainsbury, L.; Gibson, G. and Moniz-Cook, E. (1996) 'It's good to talk – man to man.' *Journal of Dementia Care, 4,* 5, Sep/Oct, 20–22.

Scheff, T.J. (1966) *Being Mentally Ill.* London: Weidenfeld and Nicolson.

Schwenk, M.A. (1981) 'Reality Orientation for the institutionalized aged: Does it help?' *Gerontologist, 19,* 373–377.

Selye, H. (1956) *The Stress of Life.* New York: McGraw-Hill.

Selye, H. (1980) 'The stress concept today.' In I. Kuthsh and L. Schlesinger (eds) *Handbook on Stress and Anxiety.* San Francisco: Josey Bass.

Sevush, S. and Leve, N. (1993) 'Denial of memory deficit in Alzheimer's disease.' *American Journal of Psychiatry, 150,* 5, 748–751.

Sherman, E. (1981) *Counselling the Ageing: An Integrative Approach.* New York: Free Press.

Shoham, H. and Neuschatz, S. (1985) 'Group therapy with senile patients.' *Social Work, 30,* 69–72.

Sillitoe, A.F. (1971) *Britain in Figures: A Handbook of Social Stastics.* Harmondsworth, Middlesex: Penguin.

Silverman, H.A. (1971) 'Excess disabilities of mentally impaired aged: Impact of individualised treatment.' *Gerontologist,* Summer, Part 1, 123–132.

Sinason, V. (1992) *Mental Handicap and the Human Condition: New Approaches from the Tavistock.* London: Free Association Books.

Sixsmith, A.; Stilwell, J. and Copeland, J. (1993) '"Rementia": Challenging the limits of dementia care.' *International Journal of Geriatric Psychiatry, 8,* 993–1000.

Smallwood, J. (1997) *Initial Report on Obtaining the Views of Activities Undertaken While in Care from People with Dementia.* Birmingham: Mental Health Services for Older Adults, Quality Department.

Snow, C.P. (1981) *The Physicists*. London: Papermac.

Social Services Inspectorate/Department of Health (1996) *Assessing Older People with Dementia in the Community: Practice Issues for Social and Health Services*. Wetherby: HMSO.

Solomon, K. and Szwarbo, P. (1992) 'Psychotherapy for patients with dementia.' In J.E. Morley, R.M. Coe, R. Strong and G.T. Grossberg (eds) *Memory Function and Aging-Related Disorders*. New York: Springer Publishing Co.

Sperlinger, D. and McAuslane, L. (1994) 'Listening to users of services for people with dementia.' *Clinical Psychology Forum, No. 73*, November, 2–4.

Starr, J.M.; Deary, I.J.; Inch, S. Cross, S. and MacLennan, W. (1997) 'Age-associated cognitive decline in healthy old people.' *Age and Ageing, 26*, 295–300.

Stengel, E. (1964) 'Psychopathology of dementia.' *Proceedings of the Royal Society of Medicine, Section of Psychiatry, 27*, October, 29–32.

Stephens, D. (1995) 'Apolipoprotein, E. and Alzheimer's Disease.' *Journal of the Royal Society for Health, 115*, 1, 4.

Stephens, L.P. (ed) (1969) *Reality Orientation: A Technique to Rehabilitate Elderly and Brain-damaged Patients with a Moderate to Severe Degree of Disorientation*. Washington D.C.: American Psychiatric Association.

Stern, Y.; Alexander, G.E.; Prohovnik, I.; Stricks, L.; Link, B.; Lennon, M.C. and Mayeux, R. (1995) 'Relationship between lifetime occupation and parietal flow – implications for a reserve against Alzheimer's disease pathology.' *Neurology, 45*, 1, 55–60.

Stokes, G. (1997) 'Reacting to a real threat.' *Journal of Dementia Care, 5*, 1, January/February, 14–15.

Stokes, G. and Goudie, F. (1990) *Working with Dementia*. Bicester, Oxon: Winslow.

Stokes, G. and Goudie, F. (1990) 'Counselling confused elderly people.' In G. Stokes and F. Goudie (eds) *Working with Dementia*. Bicester, Oxon: Winslow.

Sugarman, L. (1986) *Life-span Development*. London: Methuen.

Sutton, L. (1994) *What is it Like to Lose One's Mind* ? Paper presented at the tenth International Conference of Alzheimer's Disease International. University of Edinburgh.

Sutton, L. (1997) '"Out of the silence": When people can't talk about it.' In L. Hunt, M. Marshall and C. Rowlings (eds) *Past Trauma in Late Life*. London: Jessica Kingsley Publishers.

Sutton, L. and Cheston, R. (1997) 'Rewriting the story of dementia: A narrative approach to psychotherapy with people with dementia.' In M. Marshall (ed) *State of the Art in Dementia Care*. London: Centre for Policy on Ageing.

Sutton, L.J. and Fincham, F. (1994) 'Client's perspectives: Experiences of respite care.' *PSIGE Newsletter*, no. 49, 12–15.

Swinburn, K. and Maxim, J. (1996) 'Multi-infarct dementia – a special case for treatment?' In K. Bryan and J. Maxim (eds) *Communication Disability and the Psychiatry of Old Age*. London: Whurr.

Symonds, R.L. (1981) 'Dementia as an experience.' *Nursing Times*, September 30, 1708–1710.

Tarrier, N. and Barrowclough, C. (1990a) 'Mental health services and new research in England: Implications for community management of schizophrenia.' In A. Kales,

J. Talbot and C. Stefanis (eds) *Recent Advances in Schizophrenia.* Berlin: Springer Verlag.

Taulbee, L.R. and Folson, J.C. (1966) 'Reality Orientation for geriatric patients.' *Hospital and Community Psychiatry, 17,* 133–135.

Teri, L. and Gallagher-Thompson, D. (1991) 'Cognitive-behavioural intervention for treatment of depression in Alzheimer's patients.' *The Gerontologist, 31,* 3, 413–416.

Teri, L. and Reifler, B.V. (1987) 'Depression and dementia.' In L. Carstensen and B. Edelstein (eds) *Handbook of Clinical Gerontology.* New York: Raven Press.

Teri, L. and Wagner, A. (1992) 'Disease and depression.' *Journal of Consulting and Clinical Psychology, 4,* 60, 3, 379–391.

Terry, R. (1963) 'The fine structure of neurofibrillary tangles in Alzheimer's Disease.' *Journal of Neuropathology and Experimental Neurology, 22,* 629–642.

Thorne, B. (1992) *Carl Rogers.* London: Sage.

Thornton, S. and Brotchie, J. (1987) 'Reminiscence – a critical review of the empirical literature.' *British Journal of Clinical Psychology, 26,* 93–111.

Titmuss, R. (1997) *The Gift Relationship* (2nd edition). London: LSE Books.

Tomlinson, B.E.; Blessed, G. and Roth, M. (1968) 'Observations on the brains of non-demented old people.' *Journal of the Neurological Sciences, 7,* 331–356.

Tomlinson, B.E.; Blessed, G. and Roth, M. (1970) 'Observations on the brains of demented old people.' *Journal of the Neurological Sciences, 11,* 205–242.

Torrie, M. (1970) *Begin Again: A Book for Women Alone.* London: Dent.

Tracy, K. (1990) 'The many faces of facework.' In H. Giles and W.P. Robinson (eds) *Handbook of Language and Social Psychology.* New York: Wiley.

Truax, C.B. and Carkhuff, R.R. (1967) *Toward Effective Counselling and Psychotherapy.* Chicago: Aldine.

Twining, C. (1991) *The Memory Handbook.* Bicester, Oxon: Winslow.

Ulrich, I. (1985) 'Alzheimer changes in non-demented patients younger than sixty five: Possible early stages of Alzheimer's disease and senile dementia of the Alzheimer's type.' *Annals of Neurology,* March 17, 93, 273–277.

Unterbach, D. (1994) 'An ego function analysis for working with dementia clients.' *Journal of Gerontological Social Work, 22,* 3/4, 83–94.

Verhey, F.; Rozendaal, N.; Ponds, R. and Jolles, J. (1993) 'Dementia, awareness and depression.' *International Journal of Geriatric Psychiatry, 8,* 10, 851–856.

Viney, L.L. (1993) *Life Stories: Personal Construct Therapy with the Elderly.* Chichester: Wiley.

Vitaliano, P.P.; Young, H.M. and Russo, J. (1991) 'Burden: A review of measures used among care-givers of individuals with dementia.' *Gerontologist, 31,* 1, 67–75.

Volkow, N.R. and Tancredi, L. (1987) 'Neural substrates of violent behaviour. A preliminary study with positron emission tomography.' *British Journal of Psychiatry, 157,* 668–673.

Walker, J. and Pinhey, S. (1991) 'Elderly persons' experience of abuse.' *PSIGE Newsletter, 37,* 23–27.

Ward, L.C.; Wadsworth, A.P. and Peterson, L.P. (1994) 'Concurrent validity of measures of anxiety, depression and somatisation in elderly, demented, male patients.' *Clinical Gerontologist, 15,* 1, 3–13.

Wattis, J.P. and Hindmarch, I. (eds) (1988) *Psychological Assessment of the Elderly.* Edinburgh: Churchill Livingstone.

Weiss, R.S. (1991) 'The attachment bond in childhood and adulthood.' In C.M. Parkes, J. Stevenson-Hinde and P. Morris (eds) *Attachment Across the Life Cycle.* London: Routledge.

Welden, S. and Yesavage, J. (1982) 'Behavioural improvement with relaxation training in senile dementia.' *Clinical Gerontologist, 1,* 45–49.

Welsh, S.W., Corrigan, F.M. and Scott, M. (1996) 'Language impairment and aggression in Alzheimer's disease.' *International Journal of Geriatric Psychiatry, 11,* 257–261.

Wenger, G.C. (1994a) *Support Networks for Older People: A Guide for Practitioners.* University of Wales, Bangor: Centre for Social Policy Research and Development.

Wenger, G.C. (1994b) 'Dementia sufferers living at home.' *International Journal of Geriatric Psychiatry, 9,* 721–733.

Williams, D.D.R. and Garner, J. (1998) 'People with dementia can remember.' *British Journal of Psychiatry, 172,* 379–380.

Wilson, B.A. (1994) 'The management of memory disorders in adults.' *British Journal of Clinical Psychology, 33,* 413–415.

Wilson, B.A.; Cockburn, J. and Baddeley, A.D. (1985) *The Rivermead Behavioural Memory Test.* Bury St Edmunds: Thames Valley Test Company.

Wing, J.K. and Brown, G.W. (1970) *Institutionalism and Schizophrenia.* London: Cambridge University Press.

Winnicott, D.W. (1964) *The Child, the Family and the Outside World.* Harmondsworth, Middlesex: Penguin.

Winnicott, D.W. (1971) *Playing and Reality.* London: Tavistock.

Winnicott, D.W. (1976) *The Maturional Processes and the Facilitating Environment.* London: Hogarth Press.

Wolfensberger, W. (1972) *The Principle of Normalisation in Human Services.* Toronto: National Institute on Mental Retardation.

Wolfensberger, W. (1975) *The Origin and Nature of our Institutional Models.* Syracuse: Human Policy Press.

Wolfensberger, W. (1992) *The Principle of Normalisation in Human Services.* Syracuse: Human Policy Press.

Woods, B. (1994) 'Management of memory impairment in older people with dementia.' *International Review of Psychiatry, 6,* 153–161.

Woods, P. and Ashley, J. (1995) 'Simulated presence therapy: Using selected memories to manage problem behaviours in Alzheimer's Disease patients.' *Geriatric Nursing, 16, 1,* 9–14.

Woods, R.T. and Britton, P.G. (1985) *Clinical Psychology with the Elderly.* London: Chapman and Hall.

Woods, R.T. (1989) *Alzheimer's Disease: Coping with a Living Death.* London: Souvenir.

Woods, R.T. (1992) 'What can be learned from studies on reality orientation?' In G. Jones and B. Miesen (eds) *Care-giving in Dementia: Research and Applications.* London: Routledge.

Woods, R.T. (1994) 'Management of memory impairment in older people with dementia.' *International Review of Psychiatry, 6,* 153–161.

Woods, R.T. (1996) 'Psychological "therapies" in dementia.' In R.T. Woods (ed) *Handbook of the Clinical Psychology of Ageing.* Chichester: Wiley.

Woods, R.T. and Britton, P.G. (1985) *Clinical Psychology with the Elderly.* London: Chapman and Hall.

Worden, J.W. (1991) *Grief Counselling and Therapy,* 2nd edition. London: Tavistock/ Routledge.

World Health Organisation (1992) *The ICD-10 Classification of Mental and Behavioural Disorders: Clinical Description and Diagnostic Guidelines.* Geneva: World Health Organisation.

Wright, L.; Hickey, J.; Buckwalter, K. and Clipp, E. (1995) 'Human development in the context of aging and chronic illness: the role of attachment in Alzheimer's disease and stroke.' *International Journal of Aging and Human Development, 41,* 2, 133–150.

Wright, L.K. (1993) *Alzheimer's Disease and Marriage.* Newbury Park: Sage.

Wright, L.K. (1994) 'Alzheimer's Disease afflicted spouses who remain at home: Can human dialectics explain the findings?' *Social Science and Medicine, 38,* 8, 1037–1046.

Wright, N. and Lindesay, J. (1995) 'A survey of memory clinics in the British Isles.' *International Journal of Geriatric Psychiatry, 10,* 379–385.

Wynne, L.C.; Ryckoff, I.M.; Day, J. and Hirsch, S.I. (1958) 'Pseudo-mutuality in the family relationships of schizophrenia.' *Psychiatry, 21,* 205–220.

Yale, R. (1995) *Developing Support Groups for Individuals with Early-stage Alzheimer's Disease: Planning, Implementation and Evaluation.* Baltimore: Health Professions Press.

Yesavage, J.A.; Brink, T.L.; Rose, T.L.; Lum, O.; Huang, V.; Adey, M. and Leirer, V.O. (1983) 'Development and validation of a geriatric depression screening scale: A preliminary report.' *Journal of Psychiatric Research, 17,* 1, 37–49.

Yost, E.B.; Beutler, L.E.; Corbishley, M.A. and Allender, J.R. (1986) *Group Cognitive Therapy: A Treatment Approach for Depressed Older Adults.* New York: Pergamon.

Zarit, S.H.; Gallagher, D. and Kramer, N. (1981) 'Memory training in the community aged: Effects on depression, memory complaint, and memory performance'. *Educational Gerontology: An International Quarterly, 6,* 11–27.

Zarit, S.H. and Edwards, A.B. (1996) 'Family caregiving: Research and clinical intervention.' In R.T. Woods (ed) *Handbook of the Clinical Psychology of Ageing.* Chichester: Wiley.

NOTE: the PSIGE Newsletter that is given in a number of the references is the newsletter of the Psychologists' Special Interest Group in Elderly People. PSIGE is part of the Division of Clinical Psychology of the British Psychological Society, St Andrews House, 48 Princess Road East, Leicester LE1 7DR. www.bps.org.uk.

Index